The Natural Foods
and Nutrition Handbook

Abbreviations

Ar.	from	Arabic
Ch.	"	Chinese
D.	"	Dutch
Gk.	"	Greek
I.	"	Italian
J.	"	Japanese
L.	"	Latin
OE.	"	Old English
OF.	"	Old French
Tk.	"	Turkish

The
NATURAL
FOODS
and NUTRITION
HANDBOOK

RAFAEL MACIA

PERENNIAL LIBRARY

Harper & Row, Publishers

New York, Evanston, San Francisco, London

Contents

Abbreviations ii
Preface xiv
Cross References xv

ADDITIVES 1
ALCOHOL 4
ALFALFA 7
ANTICAKING AND FIRMING AGENTS 7
APHRODISIACS 8
BARLEY 9
BIODYNAMIC FARMING 10
BLANCHING 11
BLEACHING 11
BONE MEAL 12
BRAN 13
BREAD 13
BREWER'S YEAST 16
BUCKWHEAT 17
BULK FOOD 17

BUTTER 18

CALORIE 20

CARBOHYDRATES 21

CAROB POWDER 21

CEREAL 22

CHEESE 23

CHOCOLATE 25

CHOLESTEROL 26

CIDER 27

COFFEE 28

COLA DRINKS 30

COLORING AGENTS 32

CORN 33

DEHYDRATION 34

DESSICATED LIVER 35

DIET 35

DIGESTIVE AIDS:

  Acidophilus Preparations 37

  Enzyme Preparations 37

EGGS:

  Regular Eggs 38

  Fertile Eggs 39

ENRICHED FORTIFIED FOODS 40

ENZYMES 41

FARINA 41

FASTING 42

FATS AND OILS: 43

  Butter Oil 45

  Fish Liver Oils 46

  Garlic Oil 47

  Vegetable Oils 48

  Wheat Germ Oils 49

FLAVORING AGENTS 50

FLETCHERISM 52

FOOD ALLERGY 53

FOOD AND DRUG ADMINISTRATION 54

FOOD IRRADIATION 55

FOOD POISONING 57

FOOD SUPPLEMENTS:

  Natural 60

  Organic 60

FROZEN FOODS 61

FRUIT 62

GINSENG 64

GRAHAM FLOUR 64

GRAIN 65

HEALTH FOOD PREPARATIONS 66

HEALTH FOODS 67

HERBS 67

HERB TEAS 69

HOMINY 70

HOMOGENIZATION 71

HONEY 71

HORMONES 72

HYDROGENATION 73

JUICES:

  Fruit 74

  Vegetable 75

LACTOSE 76

LEAVENING AGENTS 77

LECITHIN 78

LIQUID FOOD 79

MACROBIOTICS 80

MALT 82

MARGARINE 82

MEAT 83

MEAT TENDERIZER 86

METABOLISM 86

MILK:
   Regular 86
   Buttermilk 88
   Certified Raw Milk 88
   Fermented Milk 90
   Goat's Milk 91

MILLET 92

MINERALS: 92
   Calcium 94
   Chlorine 95
   Copper 96
   Iodine 96
   Iron 98
   Magnesium 99
   Manganese 100
   Phosphorus 100
   Potassium 101
   Sodium 102
   Sulphur 102
   Zinc 103

MOLASSES 104

MUSHROOMS 105

NATURAL FOODS 106

NUTRIENT 106

NUTRIMENT 107

NUTRITION 107

NUTRITIONAL THERAPY 107

NUTS 108

OAT 109

ORGANIC 111

ORGANIC FARMING AND GARDENING 111

ORGANIC FOODS 112

ORGANIC PEANUT BUTTER 114

ORGAN MEATS 114

OXIDATION 115

PASTEURIZATION 116

PEANUT 116

PHOTOSYNTHESIS 117

POULTRY 118

PRESERVATIVES 120

PROTEIN 122

PROTEIN CONCENTRATE, WHOLE FISH 124

PROTEIN HYDROLYSATES 126

PROTEIN PREPARATIONS 126

RAW FOOD 127

RICE   128

ROSE HIP   129

ROYAL JELLY   130

RYE   131

SAGO   132

SAFFLOWER   133

ST. JOHN'S BREAD   133

SALT:
  Regular   134
  Sea Salt   134

SEAFOOD   135

SEAWEED: 136
  Dulse   137
  Kelp   137

SEEDS   138

SEMOLINA   139

SESAME SEEDS   140

SHORTENING   140

SORGHUM   141

SOFT DRINKS   142

SOYBEAN   143

SPICES   144

SPROUTS 145

STABILIZERS AND THICKENERS 146

STARCH 148

SUGAR:

  White Sugar 149

  Raw Sugar 151

SUN DRIED FRUITS 152

SUNFLOWER SEEDS 153

SURFACE ACTIVE AGENTS 153

TAPIOCA 154

TEA 155

TIKITIKI 157

VEGETABLE 157

VEGETARIANISM 158

VENISON 160

VITAMINS: 161

  Vitamin A 163

  Vitamin B Complex 164

  Vitamin B_1 165

  Vitamin B_2 166

  Vitamin B_8 167

  Vitamin B_{12} 168

  Niacin 169

Pantothenic Acid 170

Folic Acid 170

Para-amino-benzoic Acid **171**

Choline 171

Biotin 172

Inositol 172

Vitamin C 173

The Bioflavonoids 175

Vitamin D 176

Vitamin E 178

Vitamin K 179

Synthetic Vitamins 180

WATER:

Regular 181

Mineral 183

Spring 184

WHEAT 185

WHEAT GERM 187

WHEY 188

WHOLE FOODS 188

WILD RICE 189

YEAST 190

YOGURT 191

Preface

There is currently an enormous concern with food and nutrition, particularly a great interest in "natural" and "health" foods, not only on the part of the diet-conscious, but also on the part of the general public. However, this interest is usually associated with equally great confusion, for it is practically impossible to obtain concise and objective information in a single reference book. In many cases it is even difficult to get a clear and simple explanation of many widely used words and expressions without having to consult various technical source books.

Publications in this field are abundant. Some deal with one specific subject only, while others, attempting to encompass the entire subject matter, are usually in the nature of tracts on behalf of certain claims and convictions. Many are replete with quotations from authoritative (or claimed to be such) sources, which often contradict each other.

The purpose of this book is to present basic information about food and nutrition, especially about natural and health foods and related subjects, in an easily understandable and objective fashion. The entries here merely give the facts, explain and clarify the concepts, state the claims, and whether these claims have been substantiated by scientific evidence.

Cross References

acidophilus preparations, see: digestive aids

aromatics, see: flavoring agents, spices

arrowroot, see: sago

artesian waters, see: water

blackstrap molasses, see: molasses

brown rice, see: rice

brown sugar, see: sugar

cocoa, see: chocolate

daily recommended allowance, see: minerals, vitamins, proteins

dulse, see: seaweed

durum, see: semolina, wheat

dyes, see: coloring agents

enzyme preparations, see: digestive aids

flour, unbleached, see: bleaching

food additives, see: additives

fruitarians, see: vegetarianism

gluten bread, see: bread, semolina, wheat

hydrolized proteins, see: protein hydrolysates

kelp, see: seaweed

manioc, see: tapioca

minimum daily requirement, see: minerals, vitamins, proteins

natural honey, see: honey

natural rice, see: rice

nutritional yeast, see: brewer's yeast

oils, see: fats and oils

organic honey, see: honey

saturated fatty acids, see: fats and oils

stone ground, see: bread

trace minerals, see: minerals

truffles, see: mushrooms

unpolished rice, see: rice

unsaturated fatty acids, see: fats and oils

ADDITIVES

Substances obtained by chemical synthesis, or extracted from plant or animal sources, and mixed into or applied to various foodstuffs during manufacture or processing. Such additives serve many purposes and may be classified as Preservatives, Flavoring Agents, and Coloring Agents. Other additives are Surface Active Agents, Stabilizers and Thickeners, Anticaking Agents, Leavening Agents, and natural and synthetic supplements to enhance nutritional qualities. Many of these additives are interacting and may have more than one effect (e.g., sugar used as a flavoring agent or sweetener in jam may serve at the same time as a preservative). Often several additives are used in the same foodstuff, not only because each has a distinct effect, but also because they may complement and enhance each other's effectiveness. Many food additives have been in use for centuries (e.g., spices, gums), but the widespread use of chemical additives, and the practice of adulterating certain foodstuffs by various methods (e.g., refining, bleaching), has caused vigorous public opposition since the last century. In 1906 this opposition resulted in the passage of the first Food and Drug Law, which has been amended many times ever since. Today, all additives used by the food industry must undergo long and complicated testings, and no chemical additive can legally be used in any foodstuff until the manufacturer or processor of that particular food can prove to the Food and Drug Administration that the additive meets all the established criteria of safe usage for human consumption. At the same time, the quantity of each additive that may be safely used in foods is also determined. This quantity limit is important because not only chemicals but practically everything ingested has a "tolerance" or assimilation limit. Such limit is established either by the individual himself (e.g., too much intake of sugar, when not absorbed, may cause diarrhea in some people), or by animal experiments and testings as is the case with chemical additives. Presently, all food additives released by the Food and Drug Administration are classified as "generally recognized as safe" for their intended use; these include even salt, pepper, vinegar, baking soda, etc., that have been safely used in proper quantities for a long time. Many food additives are constantly retested in order to establish their absolute safeness for human consumption. Generally, extremely small quantities of additives are used in foods. Therefore, any possible harmful effect could only be caused by ingesting huge amounts of food at one time. Some scientists maintain that chemicals, though they may be nontoxic by scientific analysis, are not food elements. It is possible that such additives may produce, mostly through accumulation in the body, undesirable effects. Although the body is capable of coping with many, even toxic substances by detoxifying and excreting them, it is not known whether the ingestion of chemical food additives over a long period of time may or may not be detrimental to health. Practically all commercially manufactured and processed foodstuffs contain additives in order to prevent spoilage and decay, to maintain or enhance nutritional quality, to intensify flavor, and to augment or restore color, thus making them more palatable and appealing. If additives were not used at all, very few foods could be commercially produced and would be available to the public; most of them would simply cease to exist. By law, all additives used in, or applied to foods and drinks must be listed on the package or label. Sometimes, however, in order not to frighten the consumer, the names of the chemicals added to foods and drinks are abbreviated. For instance, the preservative (antioxidant) butylated hydroxyanisole is listed as "BHA," or instead of listing phenylethyl acetate on the package, it is simply stated that "artificial flavor" is added. See: **Preservatives, Flavoring Agents, Coloring Agents, Surface Active Agents, Stabilizers and Thickeners, Anticaking Agents, Leavening Agents.**

ALCOHOL (fr. Ar. *al kuhul* the powdered antimony, used as an eye cosmetic; later, the word was applied to any fine-ground substance, then it came to mean "essence," and ultimately the essential substance in alcoholic beverages)

A group of organic liquid compounds which are colorless, volatile, and flammable. Alcohols are classified according to their chemical composition, and they have different physical properties, densities, melting and boiling points. The various alcohol compounds are extensively used by many industries in the manufacture of a great variety of products from cosmetics to explosives. In common usage, the term alcohol is applied to ethyl alcohol which is the intoxicating agent in fermented and distilled beverages.

Since alcoholic beverages can occur naturally without human intervention, it is presumed that they were discovered rather than invented. Alcoholic beverages, made by fermenting cereals (beer) and the extracted juices of grapes and other fruits (wine), were already well known and produced about 5,000 years ago by the Sumerians, and approximately 3,500 years ago in Egypt and in China. Alcoholic beverages were known and widely used by later civilizations, and by many primitive societies in most parts of the ancient world. Although beer and wine were first used chiefly for religious, sacramental, and medicinal purposes, they were also drunk for pleasure. Alcohol (e.g., wine) is still part of religious ceremonies, and is also used sometimes in medicine as a cardiac stimulant in certain debilitating diseases (e.g., typhoid fever), and as a local antiseptic and astringent.

The many adverse effects of alcohol were recognized early by all cultures and societies, and warnings on the abuse of it were issued, remedies to counteract and cure those effects were prescribed, and attempts were made to regulate the production and sale of alcoholic beverages.

An Arabian alchemist, Jabir ibn Hayyan (known to the West as Geber), is credited with the invention (around 800 A.D.) of the distillation process, but it was not until the end of the thirteenth century that distilled alcohol (then called "aqua vitae" —water of life) was used as a medicine, internally and externally, mostly in small quantities. The widespread drinking of what is known today as "hard liquor" began actually around the middle of the seventeenth century when gin, whisky, and so on were invented. In the eighteenth century, sporadic protests were made against the use and abuse of alcoholic beverages, and in the nineteenth century strong temperance movements were organized in many countries. It was then suggested that the word "alcohol" may not be a derivative from the Arabic "al kuhul" but rather from "al ghul," meaning "ghost," or "evil spirit"; hence the term "spirits."

Alcohol *per se* is a narcotic poison which in larger doses affects the central nervous system (as in acute alcoholism) causing intoxication which results in muscular incoordination, uncontrollable rapid reflexes, difficulties in speech, loss of memory, delirium, and eventually coma. The regular consumption of large amounts of alcoholic beverages (chronic alcoholism) has an extremely detrimental cumulative effect upon the tissues and organs of the body (e.g., damage of the liver, pancreas and other glands, disorders of the gastrointestinal functions, mental deterioration). Because alcohol, in addition to causing loss of appetite, destroys many vital nutrients, alcoholics always suffer also from serious nutritional deficiencies. The occasional or regular moderate consumption of alcoholic beverages by a healthy person eating a balanced diet may not have any obvious effects. Response to alcohol, however, is individual and, therefore, undesirable adverse reactions may occur even after the ingestion of a small amount of alcohol. Alcoholism is now considered as a basically psychological problem (e.g., escape from reality), but alcoholism is also a nutritional disorder since alcoholics usually substitute alcohol for food. Alcohol creates what are called "empty calories," that is, the calories have no nutritional value.

ALFALFA (fr. Ar. *al-fasfasah*)

A perennial, deep-rooted leguminous plant (*Medicago sativa*), probably native to Persia, now widely grown and cultivated in Southern Europe, Asia, Argentina, and North America where it is the most important forage and hay plant. It is rich in proteins, minerals and the vitamins A, C, and E. Carotene (vitamin A) and chlorophyll are extracted from the plant for commercial use. The sprouts, especially rich in nutrients, have a subdued flavor and can be used in salads and soups. Because of their nurition value, some people recommend brewing a beverage from the leaves and stalk of alfalfa, or even chewing them raw. However, concentrated alfalfa tablets and powder for seasoning are available in health food stores. See: Sprouts.

ANTICAKING AND FIRMING AGENTS

Chemical compounds which are mixed into salt and other dried powdered food products to prevent the absorption of moisture, or added to canned vegetables and fruits in order to retain their firm texture. Salt and other pulverized food products such as puddings, instant breakfast foods, and whips easily absorb moisture from the air; this causes caking resulting in the formation of clumps. The addition of an anticaking agent (e.g., calcium phosphate, sodium silico aluminate) prevents this. In raw fruits and vegetables the naturally occurring pectin (a complex carbohydrate) keeps the cells together, but heating will usually destroy the pectin, thus causing the cooked fruits and vegetables to break up and become soft. If firming agents (e.g., calcium chloride, calcium lactate) are added, they will form with the pectin a gelatinlike substance which maintains the firmness and the structural integrity of the canned vegetables and fruits. These anticaking and firming agents must be listed on the product's package or label. See: **Additives.**

APHRODISIACS (fr. Gk. *aphrodisiakos* sexual, fr. *Aphrodite* the goddess of love and beauty in Greek mythology)

Any foodstuff or drink that allegedly arouses the sexual drive and is capable of enhancing or restoring sexual vigor and potency. Peoples of all races throughout the ages have attributed, in one form or another, aphrodisiac properties and effects to practically all foods and drinks. All such claims are based on illogical conclusions. Decrease or absence of sexual vigor and potency may be due to the lack of one or several vital and essential nutrients in the daily diet. In such cases, foods and drinks providing the required nutrients may alleviate the problem. However, since no two individuals are alike, and without first determining the nutrients lacking in the diet, the intake of any foodstuff or drink (which may be deficient in those specific nutrients) will not have the desired aphrodisiac effect. In the presence of organic lesions and ailments, or even in psychological functional disturbances, the indiscriminate consumption of food and drink having alleged aphrodisiac properties is useless and may under certain conditions be harmful.

BARLEY

An annual cereal plant (especially *Hordeum vulgare*) of the Grass family. Because of its short maturing time, barley can grow in colder regions and in high altitudes, but it cannot survive hot and humid climates. It is known to have been cultivated in ancient times in Europe, China, and Egypt. Barley was an important commodity in Europe, and its flour was used in breadmaking for many centuries. Barley is classified as winter and spring barley according to planting seasons. In the United States the production volume of barley far exceeds that of rye, but is considerably less than that of corn, wheat, and oats. It is mainly used as stock feed and as a cover crop, and only a small quantity is processed for human consumption as flour, breakfast cereal, and soup (pearl) barley. It is also used in the manufacture of malt beverages. Barley is primarily a carbohydrate food, but it offers substantial quantities of plant proteins and other nutrients.

BIODYNAMIC FARMING (fr. Gk. *bios* life and *dynamis* power)

An agronomical theory and system opposed to the use of any artificial (chemical) fertilizers, pesticides, and herbicides, and advocating the establishment of a "biological equilibrium" in the entire agriculture ("what is biologically right is economically the most profitable"); the proper utilization of the ecological relationship of various crops and vegetables ("planting wormwood between cabbages repels the flea beetle"). Introduced by the Austrian natural scientist and somewhat controversial philosopher, Dr. Rudolph Steiner (1861–1925), founder of the Anthroposophical Society, biodynamic farming immediately attracted many followers in Europe and America. Of the numerous claims made by the disciples of biodynamic farming, the most important is that plants grown by biodynamic methods have much higher nutritive values. Neither this nor many of their other claims have been proven by scientifically controlled laboratory and field tests. See: **Organic Farming and Gardening.**

BLANCHING

A name applied to several vegetable processing procedures:

(1) A process of bleaching certain vegetables (e.g., celery) without the use of chemicals simply by excluding light during the growing period. The prevention of light inhibits photosynthesis, that is, the formation of carbohydrates in the chlorophyll-containing tissues of plants. (2) Blanching is also used to remove the skin of the kernels of certain nuts (e.g., almonds) by briefly exposing the kernels to warm water or steam. (3) In canning vegetables, blanching (scalding) is used to eliminate gasses in the cell tissues, and to facilitate packaging. See: **Bleaching.**

BLEACHING

A process usually employed in the flour refining and milling industry. During the milling, the bran and the germ of the wheat grain are removed and discarded, and the remaining endosperm, consisting mainly of starch, is ground to white flour (the so-called "refined wheat flour") which is then bleached (gassed) with chlorine dioxide. Bleaching makes low grade flour "attractive" looking and also adds to the extension of its shelf life, but it destroys the few nutrients which may have been left in the flour after the refining process. Unbleached but refined flour, if not supplemented with nutrients, has not significantly more nutritional values than the bleached flour but it has a better flavor. Chemicals (e.g., sodium hypochloride) are also used in bleaching of vegetables (e.g., sprouts) to remove the chlorophyll. See: **Blanching, Coloring Agents.**

BONE MEAL

Cattle bones ground into a floury powder. It is rich in calcium, phosphorus, fluorine, and other trace minerals. Bone meal is considered to be a good food supplement, especially when a balanced calcium-phosphorus intake is desired (e.g., in deficiency cases, childhood, healing of fractures in the aged, and during pregnancy). It is available in health food stores in tablets and in powder form, and it is mixed into milk or other liquid foods.

BRAN

The outer coat covering the seed of a cereal grain as with wheat, rye, corn, rice. During the milling or polishing process, it is separated from the grain, or removed from the flour by sifting or bolting. In its inner layers, the brain contains several nutritive substances, especially vitamin B_1. The bran of various grains is used as feed for animals. For human consumption, it is produced as breakfast cereal, or it is mixed with flour in bread, not only for its nutritive values but also because its cellulose content adds roughage to the diet. See: **Bulk Food.**

BREAD

One of the oldest foods made by man requiring the combination and special preparation of various ingredients. Wheat, probably the first domesticated food plant, was known in Egypt before 5000 B.C., and the ancient Egyptians, perhaps together with the Sumerians, are credited with first making bread. (The Egyptians had some twenty varieties of bread.) As the art of breadmaking spread among the civilizations of the Mediterranean, West Asia, and Europe, bread became the most venerated food. Bread as a symbol of diligence and labor, riches and poverty, reward and punishment, the divine Providence, and of life itself, was incorporated into many languages, religious beliefs and rites.

Bread can be made from various cereal grains (wheat, rye, barley, millet, corn), and sometimes of other seeds (buckwheat). In Europe, barley flour was used for many centuries, but today wheat and rye flour are primarily used for bread and other baked products; bread baked with millet flour is common in China and India; corn flour for baking purposes is used mainly in Central America.

All cereal grains supplying flour for breadmaking contain gluten, a proteinlike substance necessary for the cohesiveness of the bread dough. (Oats do not contain gluten and therefore, oat meal is not suitable for baking bread.) The grains are ground to flour (formerly between two revolving flat round stones, today in sophisticated grinding machines), and the flour is mixed with liquid and shortening. A leavening agent is added (formerly yeast, now mostly some chemicals, such as baking soda), the dough is kneaded, shaped, allowed to rise, and then slowly baked in an oven. Before the invention of the refining and bleaching processes, bread was made with flour which was ground from whole grains. In the refining process the bran and the germ which contain the greatest amount of nutrients are separated from the endosperm of the grain and discarded (mostly used as livestock fodder). The endosperm, consisting chiefly of starch, is ground to flour. Bleaching of the flour (usually gassing it with chlorine dioxide) makes it "pure" white and enhances its keeping qualities. (Bleaching can also conceal inferior quality.) Refined and bleached flour is practically devoid of nutrients, and bread made from such flour is a pure starch food. However, most commercially processed breads are fortified and enriched with added vitamins and minerals, and sometimes with proteins. These do not, however, make it nutritionally equal to bread made from unrefined and unbleached flour. All commercial brands contain several chemical additives (e.g., preservatives, emulsifiers, leavening agents). Bread made of any whole grain flour is a wholesome food and, contrary to some beliefs, does not cause any disease. (Since it is basically a carbohydrate food, it is sometimes omitted from weight reducing diets.)

Health food stores carry a great variety of unadulterated flour (many types are stone ground) and breads made from unrefined and unbleached whole grain flour which do not contain any artificial additives. Some breads are baked with various seeds (e.g., sesame, sunflower, flax), some contain nuts, while others fruits. All these types of breads are rich in many essential nutrients.

BREWER'S YEAST (Dried Yeast; fr. OE *gist*; Gk. *zein* to boil)

The common name of a by-product obtained in the beer brewing process. Consisting largely of the dried cells of a fungus (*Saccaromyces cerevisiae*), it contains vitamin B complex, proteins (twelve of the amino acids), minerals, carbohydrates and fats. It is a concentrated source of many essential nutrients and is therefore used to some extent as a remedial agent, especially in conditions due to vitamin B deficiency. There are a variety of yeast products, several of which are not by-products of brewing but were grown in laboratories. As a food supplement, Brewer's Yeast is available in health food stores in tablet and powder form, and as soluble flakes.

BUCKWHEAT

Either one of two plants (*Fagopyrum esculeutum,* or *F. tartaricum*), members of a large family of herbs and shrubs native to Asia. Buckwheat has been cultivated and grown in Europe for centuries as a honey plant and also for its triangular seeds, which are mainly used for poultry and livestock feed. Buckwheat flour, however, is used in Russia and the Netherlands for breadmaking. The seeds contain several vitamins of the B complex (more B_1 than soybeans) and minerals, especially phosphorus. The whole grains are now utilized in breakfast cereals, or ground to flour for cooking and baking. The freshly ground flour has a distinctive taste, but the commercially marketed varieties are usually refined and mixed with other flours. Buckwheat grains and unrefined buckwheat flour are avilable in health food stores.

BULK FOOD

Fibers of uncooked foods, especially fruits and vegetables containing carbohydrates that resemble cellulose, which are not digested but, by rendering a soft bulkiness to other food material in the intestinal tracts, promote intestinal motility and absorption of more nourishment. Eating only cooked food and abstaining from raw fruits or vegetables, or taking foods in liquid form only over a long period of time (as is required in some weight reducing diets) may cause adverse reactions and become eventually a threat to health. See: Raw Food, Liquid Food, Fletcherism, Microbiotics.

BUTTER

A fatty dairy product obtained by churning the separated cream of the milk until it becomes solid. Butter was known four thousand years ago and was produced (though with very primitive methods) in many parts of the world. The milk of various animals (e.g., cow, buffalo, mare, goat, llama) was used to make butter. For a long time, however, it was used chiefly as an ointment, a medicinal remedy, an illuminating agent, and in religious services. Today butter is an important staple food in many countries and most of it is made from cow's milk. (In the United States, one-third of the milk produced is used for buttermaking.) In the dairy industry, mechanical centrifugal cream separators are used to remove the cream from the milk. The separator, made of stainless steel, is hygienic; it operates quickly and makes it possible to accurately control the fat content of the butter. Formerly, milk was set out to cool in pots and the cream which rose to the top was skimmed off. The cream was allowed to ripen by natural fermentation, and then churned into butter. After draining the butter milk, the butter was washed, sometimes salted, and battered with wooden paddles until it became a uniformly smooth mass. In the mechanized production the fermentation of the cream is usually done by inoculating it with bacteria (starter culture) and other microorganisms which cause chemical changes producing the specific butter flavor. The so-called renovated butter used in the food processing industry is made from inferior or rancid butter by melting, refining, and reprocessing it.

Butter must contain over 80 percent fat and not more than 15 percent water. The natural color of the butter is derived from carotene (the basic substance which is converted into vitamin A) present in the green plant fodder. The natural color of the butter is never deep yellow but usually whitish or pale yellow. In order to augment the natural color and to keep the tint uniform, artificial coloring agents are used, either a natural extract from the seeds of the tropical annatto tree (*Bixa orellana*), or synthetic coal-tar derivatives. (Presently, two such artificial yellow coloring agents are approved to be used in butter.) Butter is a nutritious food, it contains vitamin A, lecithin, and other growth promoting substances which are not found in oleomargarines. It has more saturated than unsaturated fatty acids but it is easily digested. Advocates of health foods recommend butter made from unpasteurized certified raw milk which is available at health food stores.

CALORIE (fr. L. *calor* heat)

As a unit measurement of heat, calorie is the amount of heat required to raise the temperature of one gram of water one degree centigrade (e.g., from 10° C to 11° C), and it is called small or gram-calorie. The measuring unit used in the study of metabolism is the large or kilo-calorie, i.e., the heat required to raise the temperature of one kilogram of water one centigrade (e.g., from 10° C to 11° C). This unit is used to express the heat-producing, or energy-producing value of food when oxidized in the body, for example, a specific food yields a certain quantity of heat energy which is stated as being so many calories. Carbohydrates (starches and sugars) such as potatoes, bread, noodles, sweets, and fats such as cream, shortenings, fatty meats, are high in calories but low in nutrients. However, carbohydrate in the form of fresh fruits, vegetables, and whole grain cereals, are low in calories but do contain the essential nutrients. The amount of calories utilized in the body depends on the individual's need for energy. Excessive (unused) calories are deposited in the form of fats in various parts of the body.

CARBOHYDRATES

These are various organic compounds consisting of carbon, hydrogen, and oxygen, most of which are formed by photosynthesis in green plants. Carbohydrates, such as sugars, starches, and celluloses, are the basic sources of food energy for men and animals, since most foods consumed consist mainly of carbohydrates. They are also involved in fat production in the body. The three main groups of carbohydrates are the simple sugars—glucose and fructose; the double sugars—sucrose, lactose, and maltose; and the multiple sugars—starches, glycogen ("animal starch"), celluloses, and dextrin (plant gum). Created through photosynthesis, the sugars are converted into starches and stored in the plants' seeds, roots, stems, and flowers. Ultimately, almost all starches will be reconverted by digestion into sugars in men and animals, and utilized as energy, or stored in the liver as glycogen for future use. Superfluous and unused carbohydrates will contribute to the build up of fat in the body. See: **Sugar, Starch, Fats and Oils.**

CAROB POWDER (fr. L. *carrubium* fr. Ar. *kharrūbah*)

The dried and then pulverized legume of a Mediterranean evergreen tree (*Ceratonia siliqua*). It contains multiple sugars (polysaccharides) which are not readily absorbed and, to a lesser degree, some vitamins and minerals. Carob powder is used chiefly as a sweetener in cooking and baking. Because of its sugar content and brownish color (not its taste), it is sometimes used as a substitute for chocolate. Candy bars and cookies made with carob powder are available in health food stores. See: St. John's Bread.

CEREAL (fr. L. Ceres the goddess of grain and agriculture in Roman mythology)

1. The generic name of plants, usually belonging to the Grass family (e.g., wheat, rice, corn, barley) yielding edible, starch-containing grains and seeds.

2. A dry food produced by special processes from grains and/or seeds. It is manufactured in various forms—flakes, kernels, globules. Some brands have added dried and sliced fruit pieces. Cereal is usually mixed into milk or cream, and eaten as a breakfast food. Since the manufacturing process requires the use of excessive heat and refining of the grains, most nutrients in the finished product are either removed or destroyed. Therefore, almost all brands of cereals are enriched to some degree with vitamins, minerals, proteins. However, many nutritionists repudiate the overemphasized nutritional values of such processed

cereals. Health food shops carry a wide variety of cereal mixtures, many with organically grown dried fruit and/or nuts, which can be eaten dry as a snack or mixed with milk.

Cereals sold in health food stores may or may not be better than those sold in regular stores. This all depends on the ingredients and the manufacturing process involved; this information is listed on the package.

CHEESE

A very nutritious food made from the milk of various animals (e.g., cow, goat, sheep). Cheese was known in many parts of the world thousands of years ago: camel's milk was used by the ancient Egyptians, goat's and sheep's milk by the early Greeks and other Mediterranean people, mare's milk by the Tartars, buffalo's milk by the people of South Asia and India, reindeer's milk by the Lapps. In the United States and Europe cow's milk is the most common source of cheese today, but goat's and sheep's milk are still used in Europe and Asia to make many popular varieties of cheese.

Cheese is made by introducing to the milk an enzyme (rennet) or lactic acid producing bacteria (or both) that curdle the protein content of the milk into a solid mass. The milk used for making cheese may be whole or skimmed, sweet or sour, and raw or pasteurized. After draining off the milk serum (whey), the cheese is allowed to ripen. This is achieved by the inherent or added microorganisms (e.g., bacteria or yeast). During this ripening and curing process, the distinctive flavor, fragrance, and texture of the cheese develop and, by enzymatic action, the milk protein is broken down into more soluble and easily digestible form.

Cheeses are classified as hard cheeses (e.g., American Cheddar, Swiss Emmental, Dutch Gouda, Italian Parmesan), semihard cheeses (e.g., French Roquefort, Italian Gorgonzola), and soft cheeses (e.g., cream and cottage cheeses, Belgian Limburger, French Brie). Processed cheese, a blend of different varieties, ground, melted, and mixed with gelatin and water, is usually homogenized and pasteurized. It contains far less nutrients than the other types of cheeses. All the natural cheeses (as opposed to the processed cheeses) are an excellent source of complete proteins, minerals (e.g., calcium, phosphorus, iron, sulphur) and, if made of whole milk, of vitamin A. (Two tablespoons of cottage cheese have the same complete protein value as one ounce of meat.)

CHOCOLATE (fr. Aztec *xocoatl*, fr. *cacahuatl* cocoa beans)

An aromatic and nourishing preparation made from the seeds (beans) of the cacao or chocolate tree (*Theobroma cacao*) widely used as a beverage, confectionery, and as a flavoring ingredient in baking and cooking. The cacao tree is native to tropical South and Central America where it was first cultivated by the Indians. The chocolate beverage made from the beans was especially highly valued by the Aztecs, and was introduced to Europe by the Spanish in the seventeenth century; it quickly became a fashionable drink in most Western European countries.

The cacao seeds are enclosed in the fruit (pod) which is fermented by naturally occurring yeast and bacteria to eliminate the bitter taste due to the slight caffeine (theobromine) content of the seeds. The cured and roasted clean seeds, the "cocoa nibs," are the basic raw material from which various products are manufactured. The beans are rich in fat (the so-called cocoa butter) which is extracted by pressure and used by the food, pharmaceutical, and cosmetic industries. Cocoa used for beverage and flavoring is the powder of the finely ground fat-free beans, while chocolate is a product which contains the cocoa butter. Chocolate manufacturing, a complex process requiring special machinery, started in the last quarter of the nineteenth century when the process of blending the beans with sugar and condensed milk was invented. It developed into a commercially important industry, particularly in Switzerland, the Netherlands, the United States, and Germany. The cocoa beans are rich in carbohydrates and proteins, and their fat content is high in unsaturated fatty acids. Both the cocoa beverage and chocolate have good nutritive values. There are some claims that cocoa and chocolate (and products containing them) prevent the assimilation of calcium and may have undue stimulating effects. Neither claim has been substantiated by medical evidence. Consumption of chocolate, however, is usually not recommended for obese persons or for those who tend to gain weight.

CHOLESTEROL (fr. Gk. *chole* bile and *stereos* solid) A complex, fatlike substance, present to some extent in all tissues of the body (but especially in human and animal fats and oils), in the brain, liver, and kidney, in the blood and bile, in milk and eggs, and in some endocrine glands. Cholesterol has been shown experimentally to be a major factor causing, or worsening, various cardio-vascular diseases. It is, however, an essential substance in the physiological processes and cannot completely be eliminated from the body. It has been proven that a diet rich in saturated fats (found mainly in animal and certain dairy products) will cause an elevation of blood cholesterol, while a diet containing mainly unsaturated fats (found chiefly in vegetables and fish) will lower the blood cholesterol level. However, the body manufactures cholesterol regardless of whether it has been excluded from the diet; it is also able to convert vegetable fats into animal type fats and produce cholesterol from starch and sugar. Under certain conditions, blood cholesterol may rise even if the diet is low in animal fats; furthermore, a decrease in blood cholesterol does not necessarily mean a decrease of the cholesterol in the tissues. See: **Fats and Oils.**

CIDER

In the United States the name generally applies to commercially processed apple juice. The apples are grated in special mills and the juice extracted. (Cider is also made from pears and it is called "perry.") The commercially produced cider is usually pasteurized, or artificial preservatives are added to it, and occasionally it is sweetened with sugar. Some cider brands are blended in order to augment the balance between the sugar, malic and tannic acids, the main components of cider. Apple cider (also called sweet cider) is the traditional beverage served with Thanksgiving dinner in the New England states. Fermented apple juice (called "hard" cider) contains alcohol and is more popular in various European countries (Germany, Austria, Switzerland) than in the United States. Cider is sometimes confused with must, a beverage obtained during wine-making from the juice of grapes before completion of the fermentation process. (Must contains alcohol and is popular in most wine-producing regions.) Fresh apple juice, as all fruit juices, contains various vitamins, minerals, enzymes, fruit acids, and is a nutritive drink. The nutritional value of the commercially manufactured cider depends on the process employed in its productions. See: **Fruit Juices.**

COFFEE

The name of a beverage made from the seeds (beans) of closely related evergreen shrubs (*Coffea arabica, C. robusta, C. liberica*). It was probably native to Ethiopia (known before 1000 A.D.) where it was made to a pulp mixed with fat for food, and the pods fermented to produce an alcoholic beverage. Coffee is now cultivated in nearly all tropical regions. Coffee as it is known today was invented by the Arabs who introduced it to other countries of the Near East from where, in the seventeenth century, it reached Europe. By the end of that century, coffee became known in North America, and about the same time the Spanish planted the first coffee shrubs in their South American colonies. In North America, coffee as a beverage became really popular only after the Boston Tea Party (1773).

Coffee is prepared in various ways in different countries:

"Turkish" coffee is made from the finely pulverized roasted beans with honey or sugar added; the Italian "espresso" is made from the almost charred beans by pressing steam through the ground mass. In the United States and in Europe, coffee is usually prepared by filtering or simply boiling the roasted and ground beans. Because of the invigorating effect and pleasant aroma from its volatile oils, coffee is a widely used beverage in most countries. It contains caffeine, a slightly bitter crystalline substance which, if taken in moderation, is a mild stimulant to the nervous and cardiovascular systems. Caffeine preparations are used sometimes for certain heart conditions, migraine headaches, and opium poisoning. However, caffeine is a diuretic (it increases the excretion of urine) and it retards the elimination of tissue wastes. There are several brands of coffees available from which the caffeine has been removed without significantly affecting the aroma.

In moderate amounts, coffee is generally regarded as harmless for a healthy person. In some people, however, even one or two cups of coffee may lead to insomnia, nervousness, and excessive urination. There are many ailments (e.g., high blood pressure, various heart diseases, stomach ulcers) toward which coffee may be very harmful. It is also not recommended for growing children. The raw coffee bean, as all seeds, contains certain nutrients but through roasting and boiling of the bean, they are completely destroyed; therefore, coffee has no nutritional values. See: **Tea, Chocolate, Cola Drinks.**

COLA DRINKS

A mixture of carbonated water and, chiefly, extracts from coca leaves and kola (cola) nuts, with sugar, caramel, some acid, and aromatic substances added. Coca (not to be confused with cacao) is the name of various South American shrubs, particularly the *Erthroxylon coca*, from which most cocaine is derived. (Cocaine is a highly habit forming drug, and its continued use may lead to a complete deterioration of the nervous system. In medicine, it is used mainly as a local anesthetic.) Chewing of the tealike, dried leaves of the coca shrub has been practiced for centuries by South American Indians. The effects usually depend on

the amount of and the length of time the leaves
are chewed. A small amount chewed for a short
time has a stimulating, or even excitatory, effect,
while chewing for a longer time causes a slow-
down in mental and physical activities and also
drowsiness. The kola nut (also called the gourou-
nut) is the bitter tasting, caffeine-containing seed
in the pod of kola trees, especially of the *Cola
nitida,* native to Africa but now cultivated also in
other tropical areas. Extractions from the kola nut
are used in various cardiac and nerve stimulating
drugs. The nuts are chewed for their stimulating
effect by the native population in various parts of
Africa. Listing of the exact quantities of the coca
and kola extracts used in the manufacture of the
various soft drinks ("soft" means that they do not
contain alcohol) is not required by law. Many
physicians maintain that imbibing drinks containing kola and coca can become a habit just as with
coffee drinking, and most physicians, nutritionists,
and dentists warn of the numerous deleterious
effects of such drinks to the nervous and digestive
systems as well as to the teeth. They recommend
a very moderate intake, or particularly for children, the complete elimination of these drinks
from the diet. They have no nutritional values.
See: **Soft Drinks.**

COLORING AGENTS (Dyes)

Soluble or insoluble materials obtained by chemical synthesis, or extracted from natural sources (plants, animals), and mixed into, or applied to various foodstuffs in order to retain, enhance, or recreate the natural color and appearance particular to certain foods and drinks. Coloring agents have no preservative properties, and contribute no flavors or nutritional values, but are considered as necessary food additives because people usually have a preconceived image of the appearance and color of most foods and drinks (yellow butter, red meat). Because during the manufacturing process the original or natural color of many foods changes, a great variety of commercially produced foods and drinks contain coloring agents. For instance, a yellow color, obtained from natural sources, is used in butter, margarine, and oils, while a synthetized red dye is used in soft drinks and meat products. Using coloring agents to conceal inferior products (e.g., gassing unripe tomatoes with ethylene to produce a red color) is illegal. There are many natural coloring agents available but the ten synthetic water-soluble dyes approved for use by the food industry account for approximately 90 percent of all coloring agents added to foods and drinks. Synthetic dyes are less expensive than natural coloring agents, are more uniform and stable, and provide more intense colors. As with all other food additives, coloring agents used must be stated on the product's package or label. See: **Additives.**

CORN

A tall, annual cereal (grain) plant (*Zea mays*) of the Grass family, bearing seeds on elongated ears. (Actually, corn is the name given to the leading cereal crop in any particular country: in England it is wheat, in Ireland oats, in the Americas and Australia the Indian corn or *maize*.) Corn has been domesticated and cultivated in many varieties (sweet corn, corn for meal, popcorn) by the Indians since ancient times. It is the result of the cross-breeding of various related plants, and it has been so completely adapted to cultivation that it never reverts to its ancestral wild form. Corn as we know today cannot grow wild, and requires man's care. From America, corn was introduced to other parts of the world and is now widely distributed and cultivated as an important agricultural product in many countries, especially in Eastern Europe, the USSR, and Australia. Because it was possible to grow various distinct and easily identifiable strains of corn (e.g., yellow, red, white), corn became in the early part of this century the subject of extensive and revolutionary scientific experiments. These efforts resulted in the development of a hybrid corn which produces a greater yield and contains more sugar and less starch. It is also more uniform and can be bred to specifications. Today, these hybrid seeds are used for practically all commercially grown types of corn and the production of hybrid corn seeds has become a large industry. In the United States (the world's largest producer) corn is used primarily as feed grain for animals. In Central America, however, corn is still an important staple food and corn flour (meal) is widely used in baking and cooking. Products extracted from corn (oil, starch, sugar) are used in various industries. Generally, in human nutrition the role of corn is not significant. It is consumed boiled or cooked as a side dish, sometimes mixed with vegetables, or freshly roasted as popcorn. Several baked products contain corn meal, and various breakfast cereals are made from corn. Corn oil is used extensively in the manufacture of margarine. It has about the same unsaturated fatty acid content as soybean and sunflower oil. See subentry on Vegetable Oils under **Fats and Oils, Hominy.**

DEHYDRATION

A process whereby the water content of certain foods is removed through evaporation in the presence of hot air. The heat used in the process destroys some of the nutrients, while the contact with air oxidizes others.

DESICCATED LIVER (fr. L. *desiccare* to dry, fr. L. *siccus* dry)

Liver is one of the most complete and potent single source of many important nutrients. Desiccation is a process whereby the liver, after removal of the lining, the connective tissues and the external fat, is slowly dried at low temperature in a vacuum chamber, thus preserving all vital nutrients. Desiccated liver is a very rich concentrated source of iron, protein (with all the essential amino acids), the vitamin B complex and, to a lesser degree, the vitamins A, C, and D. In order to get these benefits, it is popular as a food supplement with vegetarians and other people who for some reason abstain from eating meat products. Desiccated liver is available in health food stores in tablets, capsules, and in powder form.

DIET (fr. L. *diaeta*, fr. Gk. *diaita* lit. manner of living)

1. The food and drink regularly and customarily consumed.

2. A particular prescribed course, including amount and preparation, of selected solid and liquid foods and food supplements for the purpose of (a) preventing or correcting nutritional deficiencies (in case of calcium and phosphorus deficiency, a diet is prescribed containing mostly milk, yellow cheeses, egg, and poultry); (b) attaining in certain illnesses a therapeutically necessary and effective balance of the nutrients (a bland diet, containing the necessary nutrients but free of irritating foods and spices, is given to patients with stomach ulcers), or eliminating certain foods from the diet which may have adverse effects or aggravate the disease (salt-free diet in certain heart conditions); (c) reducing weight (low-calorie diet usually containing 1,200 calories or less and consisting mainly of high-protein foods and excluding fats and carbohydrates), or gaining weight (high-calorie diet usually containing 4,000 calories or more a day and consisting of foods rich in fats, carbohydrates, and proteins).

In addition, there are a great variety of diets which may be prescribed temporarily for acute conditions (apple diet: grated apple used in the treatment of infantile diarrhea), or chronic diseases (diabetic diet excluding ordinary sugar and starchy foods).

The need for, and the ingredients of, any special diet for any reason can be determined only by a thorough physical examination and should always be carried out under the supervision of a physician.

DIGESTIVE AIDS:

Acidophilus Preparations (fr. L. *acidus* acid, and fr. Gk. *philein* to love)

The term acidophilus is applied to microorganisms (family *Lactobacteriaceae*) which thrive in highly acid media and which, by fermenting carbohydrates such as lactose (milk sugar), produce lactic acid and often gas (carbon dioxide). Lactic acid helps in the absorption and assimilation of the nutrients in the intestine and retards the growth of putrefactive organisms. Acidophilus preparations are paramedical products, used as digestive aids, containing usually one or several strains of the microorganism, e.g., *Lactobacillus acidophilus*, *L. bulgaricus* (used in making yogurt), *L. caucasicus* (found in certain grains). Some products contain in addition carbohydrates (e.g., pectin) derived from fruits that produce other organic acids which are also beneficial to the intestinal flora. Acidophilus preparations are available at health food stores either in powder or in carbonated liquid form, and as wafers.

Enzyme Preparations

Paramedical products used to intensify and facilitate the digestive process. They are usually composed of various enzymes active in the conversion and absorption of the nutrients in the alimentary tract, for example, amylase (converts starch into sugar), pancreatin (a substance, secreted by the pancreas, containing four principal digestive enzymes), papain (derived from the papaya fruit, it converts protein into amino acids). Some preparations also contain several acids, for example, glutamic acid (obtained by the decomposition of proteins), taurocholic acid (obtained from the bile), which serve as additional digestive aids. Enzyme preparations in tablet form, and as chewing gum, are available at health food stores.

EGGS

Regular Eggs

In biology, the female sex cell which, after fertilization by the male sperm, can develop into a new living being capable of independent existence. In common usage, the term is applied to the hard-shelled egg produced by birds, especially by domestic poultry. Within the egg are all the essential nutritive materials necessary for the complete development of the young (chick), without the need of anything from the environment except oxygen (air can penetrate the porous egg shell). The egg consists of the calcium-rich protective hard shell, the inner and outer lining membranes within the shell enclosing the egg white (albumin), which in turn contains the yolk attached by a pair of spiral bands to the opposite ends of the lining membranes.

Eggs are a very rich and concentrated source of many nutrients, especially of biologically highly effective proteins, of the vitamins A, B_2, B_6, and the other members of the B complex (niacin, choline, pantothenic acid, folic acid, B_1, inositol, and biotin), and vitamin D, as well as the minerals phosphorus, iron, sulphur, copper, manganese, and magnesium. Though eggs are rich in cholesterol they contain lecithin which in combination with choline and inositol prevent cholesterol from being deposited in the blood vessels and the liver by keeping it solvent and by augmenting its metabolism.

Eggs may be consumed in any form (raw, boiled, fried, baked), alone or together with many other foods. It is, however, not advisable to eat raw egg white alone without the yolk because the white contains avidin, a protein which destroys biotin, the vital growth-vitamin. The yolk contains substances which prevent this and, in addition, supplies biotin.

Fertile Eggs (also called "Organic Eggs")

These eggs are produced by hens bred on organic farms, and allowed to freely mate with the rooster. While hens kept in chicken coops are usually given commercially processed feed, hens raised in freedom will choose and pick any food they find on the ground. Advocates of fertile eggs claim that such eggs contain more vitamins (especially B_{12}), and other nutrients, and are richer in hormones. Apart from the fact that the requirement for chicken hormones in humans has never been established, these claims have not been substantiated by evidence. The highly nutritious commercially processed chicken feed sometimes contains fish meal that may be tasted in the eggs. Therefore, fertile or organic eggs may have a better, more "natural" taste. See: **Organic Foods.**

ENRICHED, FORTIFIED FOODS

The commercial processing of foodstuffs (precooking, pasteurizing, refining, milling, bleaching) usually destroys, partially or entirely, all or several of their intrinsic nutrients and other vital substances. In order to replace them, synthetized nutrients are added to the foodstuffs. It must be noted, however, that such replacement is not always feasible and does not restore in every instance the destroyed, decreased, or changed nutritive values. Certain foods, even though their nutrients have not been removed or destroyed, are supplemented with additional nutrients in order to intensify the nutritional values (e.g., whole wheat bread is fortified with wheat germ). It is also customary to add synthetic nutrients to edible or drinkable material made almost exclusively from chemicals as in the addition of vitamin C to a powder made with artificial flavoring and sweetening agents that, dissolved in water, will produce a drink. See: **Natural Foods, Natural Food Supplement.**

ENZYMES (fr. Gk. *enzyme* leaven)

Any of the numerous complex organic substances, mostly proteins or similar to proteins, that are produced by living cells. By facilitating or accelerating catalytic actions, enzymes govern all chemical reactions and transformations in the body and are, therefore, essential for the breakdown in the digestion, assimilation, and utilization of all nutrients. The formation and activity of the enzymes within the body are interdependent with those of the proteins, vitamins, and minerals. Although enzymes perform within and at the intrinsic temperature of the organisms (animals, plants), they are available only in raw, uncooked foods, as their effectiveness is destroyed by heat.

FARINA (fr. L. flour, meal, fr. L. *far* a wheat species)

A floury substance usually made from wheat (durum) after the removal of the germ and bran.

It is almost pure starch, therefore most farina products are enriched with added vitamins and minerals. Farina is sometimes used in the commercial manufacture of noodles, but it is chiefly eaten as a breakfast cereal cooked in milk.

FASTING (the complete abstinence from food and drinks; med.: "absolute diet")

Fasting has been popular in varying degrees among the peoples of all races. It has been incorporated into the dietary laws of several religions and religious sects. It is also sometimes used as a form of protest against, or for, various causes (e.g., hunger strike in a prison).

While many benefits are claimed for temporary or prolonged fasting ("it purifies the body," "it enlightens the mind,") there is no medical evidence that it has any therapeutic value. (Fasting should not be confused with the temporary restriction or complete elimination of certain foods and drinks in special corrective diets.) Many cases have been reported of the survival of people who completely abstained from all solid foods for a relatively long period of time. However, in such cases certain liquid foods (e.g., fruit juices) and water were consumed. During the fasting process the human body uses its own stored nutritional resources. But without liquid intake the survival period would be very short.

Prolonged fasting can be very detrimental to one's health. Depriving the body of essential nutrients will not only cause debilitation but in most cases, irreversible damages. Complete abstinence from food for any length of time and for any reason (e.g., "starvation diet" for weight reduction) should be carried out only at the recommendation and under the strict supervision of a physician. See: **Diet.**

FATS AND OILS

General

Organic substances similar to carbohydrates that are derived from animal or plant sources. They occur mostly combined with proteins or carbohydrates. Fats and oils are compounds of carbon, hydrogen, and oxygen, having less oxygen than carbohydrates. At room temperature, the fats are usually solid and the oils liquid. Chemically, fats and oils are *saturated* or *unsaturated* fatty acids.

Fats and oils are an important part of the diet. In nutrition, they provide building material for the tissues of the body, and release more energy than the other nutrients. Fat supports the internal organs; it forms a protective cushion around the nerves, and protects the body against changes in temperature. Fats are the natural carriers and protectors of the fat-soluble vitamins A, D, E, and K, and also help in the utilization of the hormones.

The metabolism of fats, however, is still not fully understood. It is known that the body requires both types of fats, the saturated and the unsaturated ones. The saturated fatty acids (having more hydrogen) are more slowly absorbed than the unsaturated fatty acids. The latter are very efficacious in minute quantities and are considered essential for good health (therefore sometimes referred to as "vitamin F"); they are also needed for the utilization of the saturated fatty acids and for the diffusion of calcium from the blood into the tissues. The unsaturated fatty acids are the linoleic, linolenic, and arachidonic, of which the linoleic acid is the most important, although the arachidonic acid is believed to be more effective in promoting growth.

When exposed to air, fats and oils tend to oxidize quickly, thus becoming rancid. Rancidity destroys the vitamin E, and disturbs the assimilation of other fat-soluble vitamins. Commercial processing and heating have, to a certain degree, similar effects on these vitamins, especially on vitamin E. Unsaturated fatty acids contain naturally occurring substances (antioxidants) which prevent serious losses of the fat-soluble vitamins, but only wheat germ and cottonseed oils are sufficiently protected against the destruction of vitamin E caused either by oxidation or excessive heating.

Over-heating fats and oils, especially during frying, will not only reduce the intrinsic nutritive values, but will also decompose them and produce a highly irritating substance which has been shown to cause cancer in experimental animals. Fats and oils should be quickly heated to the degree below the temperature of decomposition. Oils and shortenings tolerate the greatest heat, up to 450° F, without decomposing; lard up to 430° F; butter up to 406° F; and olive oil up to 347° F.

Fats of land animals and animal products contain more saturated and less unsaturated fatty acids than fish, shellfish, and vegetable oils. Saturated fatty acids have been found in many cases to raise the cholesterol level in the blood and probably contribute to the incidence of certain cardiovascular diseases.

The excessive intake of fats and oils, regardless of their saturated or unsaturated fatty acid content, will retard digestion and result in undesirable fatty deposits in the body, causing susceptibility to heart ailments and other degenerative diseases. On the other hand, complete elimination of fats from the diet will deprive the body of necessary nourishment, disrupt the absorption and utilization of many nutrients, and result in severe disorders.

Butter Oil (butter fat)

A pure oil made by melting and boiling butter in order to evaporate the water content, and then straining it to remove the solid residues. Butter oil has good cooking and keeping qualities; it remains fresh in covered containers for many months. Butter oil (also called "clarified butter") is manufactured in large quantities, sometimes with spices and fragrances added, in India and the Middle East, especially in Egypt. In India (made from cow or buffalo milk) it is called "ghee," and is widely used in cooking, baking, and as a seasoning. Ghee has been known since ancient times and was (and still is) used as a medicinal remedy, and as a highly venerated sacrificial oil in the practice of Hinduism.

Fish Liver Oils

A yellowish oil obtained from the liver of various fish, particularly the codfish (*Gadus morrhua*). People living in the northern latitudes, close to, or in the arctic regions having little vegetation and sunshine, observed centuries ago that consumption of fish liver had greatly beneficial effects, especially for growing children. Later it was discovered that the oil contained in the liver is very rich in the vitamins D and A, and also contains small amounts of minerals (e.g., phosphorus, iodine, sulphur). Vitamin D is essential for the assimilation of phosphorus and calcium, thus it is a major factor in the development and maintenance of healthy bones and teeth. Vitamin D is formed in the skin by exposure to sunshine and there is actually no natural food that is an adequate source of it. Vitamin A, equally important, is found in plant products only in the form of its precursor carotene which is converted in the liver into true vitamin A. Fish liver oils are the only concentrated natural food sources of vitamin D and true vitamin A. Although both vitamins A and D have been synthetized, health food advocates and some nutritionists recommend supplementing the diet with natural fish liver oil derivatives. Health food stores carry various concentrated fish liver oils in capsule and liquid form.

Garlic Oil

Garlic (*Allium sativum*), a relative of the onion, is a perennial plant of the Lily family. Its edible bulb, consisting of cloves, is rich in sugar and a pungent oil, and is used in cooking as a flavoring agent. It is especially popular in the Mediterranean countries and the Orient. Garlic oil, because of the inherent enzymes, is a digestive stimulant and has been used as such since ancient times. It helps to expel gas from the alimentary canal, thus relieving intestinal discomfort. However, the many other medicinal properties and wondrous effects attributed to garlic and its oil are unfounded. It neither prevents nor cures diseases, nor is it an aphrodisiac or a rejuvenating agent. (Garlic oil and powder have been found to have certain bactericidal and fungicidal properties when used on microorganisms which cause diseases in plants.) Deodorized garlic oil, alone or with added oil of the parsley seed, in capsules or tablet form, and garlic powder for seasoning, are available in health food stores.

Vegetable Oils

Since natural vegetable oils are rich in unsaturated fatty acids, they are preferred to animal fats by those who wish to decrease or eliminate an additional build-up of cholesterol in the body. Vegetable fats are prone to rancidity which destroys their vitamin E content. Because fats are stored in the cells of the body, this may, similar to rancidity, also have a destructive effect on the vitamin E complex. Of the popular vegetable oils only the cottonseed and wheat germ oils are self-protected against the antivitamin E action of the unsaturated fatty acids by having adequate supplies of the vitamin E complex.

Safflower oil contains the highest amount (80–90 percent) of all the unsaturated fatty acids, and 70–80 percent of the linoleic acid, the most important fatty acid.

Corn, soybean, sesame, and sunflower oils have about the same total fatty acid content (around 80 percent), while corn, soybean, and sunflower oils contain about 50–60 percent of the linoleic acid; sesame oil has approximately 70 percent of it.

Cottonseed and peanut oil have over 70 percent

of the total unsaturated fatty acids, and 30–50 percent of the linoleic acid.

The manufacturing methods in extracting vegetable oils may involve either a heating process which will decrease or destroy the nutrients in the oils, or a mechanical "cold-extraction" process whereby heat is not used, thus preserving the nutritional values. Cold-extracted vegetable oils are recommended by health food advocates for use in cooking (cooking, however, reduces the nutrients), in salads, or added to other foods. Cold-extracted vegetable oils are available in vacuum-sealed jars or cans (which should always be kept tightly closed and refrigerated) at health food stores and better groceries. See also: **Hydrogenation, Margarine.**

Wheat Germ Oil

Extracted from its natural source, the wheat germ, it contains all the active principles of the vitamin E complex, that is, the alpha, beta, gamma, and delta tocopherol, in higher concentration than any other vegetable oil. It also contains vitamins of the B complex, vitamin A, and unsaturated fatty acids. As a food supplement, wheat germ oil is usually used in salads or added to other foods, rather than for cooking or frying. Health food stores carry freshly pressed and unadulterated wheat germ oil in vacuum-packed cans and bottles which must be kept tightly covered and refrigerated. Wheat germ oil as well as the vitamin E complex, distilled from unrefined and cold-extracted vegetable oils, are also available in capsules. See: **Wheat Germ.**

FLAVORING AGENTS

Materials obtained by chemical synthesis or by extraction from natural sources, and added to various foods and drinks in order to create, enhance, modify, or, in some cases, mask the natural flavor (taste) or fragrance (odor) particular to certain foodstuffs. The use of spices, herbs, and salt for seasoning and flavoring food to make it more appealing has been used by all people since ancient times. Many natural flavoring agents are available, but synthetic flavors are preferred by the food industry because they are less expensive, can be manufactured uniformly, and are not dependent on the seasons, climate, and soil, as with some natural sources. The largest group of flavorings used today in foods consists of essential oils.

Flavor enhancers are substances which do not have an inherent flavor but when added to various foods will intensify the natural taste, especially of those foods which have a high protein content. The most widely used flavor enhancer (or potentiator) is monosodium glutamate (MSG). There are three additional flavor potentiators approved of and used in soft drinks, cereals, vegetable, fruit, and other commercially processed products. Natural and artificial sweeteners are considered as flavoring agents since they constitute the basic taste of many foods and drinks. The natural sweeteners, such as sugar and honey, also contribute in many cases a certain fullness to foods and drinks, and may even act, to varying degrees, as preservatives. Saccharin, the artificial sweetener, discovered in 1879 and first commercially produced in 1900, is a colorless and odorless crystalline powder. It is approximately 500 times sweeter than sugar. Because it is not sugar and contains no calories, it is widely used whenever the intake of sugar is contraindicated (e.g., in diabetic conditions, in weight reducing). Cyclamate compounds, approximately 30 to 50 times sweeter than sugar, were discovered in 1937, and first introduced commercially in 1950 under the trade name "Sucaryl" (calcium cyclamate). When in 1969 it was discovered that they caused certain adverse effects in experimental animals, cyclamate production was halted, but new and extensive laboratory testings were resumed in 1970.

Several acids are added to a great variety of foods and drinks to intensify or supplement the flavor and provide tartness. These are called "fruit acids" because originally they were extracted from various fruits. As flavoring agents or flavor enhancers, they are used mainly in products containing fruits or fruit derivatives. In other foodstuffs, such as processed cheeses, cheese spreads, and dips, these acids help to provide the desired tartness and texture. Of all the acids used in foods and drinks, citric acid accounts for more than half. Alkalis (e.g., sodium carbonate, ammonium bicarbonate), opposite compounds to acids, are used to prevent foods from becoming too acid. Controlling acidity can also augment flavor in many cases. The use of flavoring agents and enhancers, the addition of acids, alkalis, and sweeteners, including sugar, must be stated on the product's package or label. See: Additives.

FLETCHERISM

The theory, introduced by the American nutrition writer, Horace Fletcher (1849–1919), according to which good digestion and proper utilization of all nutrients can only be attained if every bit of food is chewed thoroughly (thirty to seventy times) and is in a liquid state before being swallowed. Even liquid foods (milk, soup) should be rolled around in the mouth until they are well-mixed with saliva. Fletcherism was quite popular in the first decades of this century. Today, it is known that the body is able to digest proteins without much chewing, and most proteins will be digested better if swallowed in compact pieces rather than chewed to a pulp. Although starchy foods require more chewing in order to be mixed with ptyalin (predigestive enzyme in the saliva), liquefying them by overchewing is neither beneficial nor necessary. See: Macrobiotics.

FOOD ALLERGY (fr. Gk. *allos* other and *ergon* work)

A condition caused by a specific reaction in some people to certain substances in foods that, in similar amounts, do not have the same effect on others. These substances are called allergens or antigens. The term allergy is applied to all types of human hypersensitivity, such as exaggerated or unusual bodily reaction to physical agents (cold, light, heat), to air-borne substances (pollens, fumes, dust), to certain microorganisms (parasites, bacteria, fungi), to contactants (chemicals, hair, certain fabrics), and to drugs (penicillin, aspirin). An allergy may be hereditary or psychological, that is, the condition resembles allergy but it is due to the mental or emotional state of the person.

A great variety of foods cause allergic reactions of different degrees in many people. Most common are reactions to certain fruits (strawberries, citrus fruits), to fats and oils (milk fat, oil in salad dressings), to spices (mustard, horseradish), and to such foods as eggs, chocolate, certain seafoods and so on. Some people have an unusual sensitivity to ordinary food proteins, in which case "predigested" proteins (protein hydrolysates) are used in the diet. Allergic reactions to foods may manifest themselves in gastrointestinal disturbances (nausea, vomiting, diarrhea), in effects on the skin (rashes, acne), in "hot flashes," in respiratory difficulties. Treatment of allergy usually consists of injecting the causing agent (allergen) thereby producing a deliberate reaction which results in the "desensitization" of the person. In some cases, certain drugs (antihistamine) are used to alleviate the symptoms. If feasible, abstaining from the foods which cause the reaction is the best way to prevent food allergy.

FOOD AND DRUG ADMINISTRATION

The United States Food and Drug Administration (FDA), headed by an appointed Commissioner, is a federal agency within the Department of Health, Education, and Welfare. It has several divisions and branches staffed by qualified scientists and technicians (e.g., Division of Food, Toxicity Branch), and its own testing laboratories and field investigators.

The FDA is charged with the administration of the Food, Drug, and Cosmetic Act, which was enacted in 1938 (and amended many times since) and superseded the Pure Food and Drug Act of 1906. The food laws define the criteria for the

wholesomeness and purity of all foodstuffs, and
regulate their manufacture and processing, including quality, weight, use and quantity of additives
(no chemical can legally be used until the manufacturer proves to the FDA that it is safe for
human consumption), packaging, labeling, distribution and so on. The FDA is responsible for
enforcing the law by supervising manufacturing
methods, inspecting manufacturing and processing
facilities, systematically testing the food products
sold to the consumer, formulating standards and
definitions for truthful labeling. FDA investigators
have the authority to seize and confiscate foods
found to be deleterious to health, or which otherwise do not conform to the law. If warranted, the
FDA can request changes in manufacturing processes, discontinuation of products, and even the
closing of manufacturing, processing, and other
food handling facilities. The laws provide penal-
ties for any violation of the Food, Drug, and Cosmetic Act.

FOOD IRRADIATION

The possibility of preserving food by radiation was
recognized in the first decades of this century, and
in the mid-1940s investigations began to determine
the methods, processes, and problems involved.
But it was not until the early 1950s that large-scale
research was undertaken and results achieved.

In the radiation process the food is exposed mostly to cobalt-60 (a radioactive chemical element produced in nuclear reactors) emitting rays (e.g., gamma rays) which penetrate the food, thereby causing changes in the atoms ("ionizing the food atoms") and, depending on the dosage applied, either destroy or inhibit the growth of decay-causing microorganisms. Some of the tissue cells of the irradiated food are also destroyed or altered, but without harmful effects to the food; the irradiated food does *not* become radioactive.

Food preservation by low dosage radiation is equivalent to pasteurization. Sterilization is accomplished by high dosage. With low dosage there is less loss of vitamins than in canning, freezing, or drying. As with most other preservation processes, radiation does affect the appearance and, in some cases, the taste, odor, and color of certain foods. Since no other method (with or without chemicals) can preserve fresh or precooked food for a comparable length of time, the feasibility and the techniques of irradiation are being studied and pursued in many countries more thoroughly and more extensively than any other food processing method.

In the United States most of this research is being carried out by the Army in cooperation with many scientific institutions under the aegis of the U.S. Atomic Energy Commission, though only the Food and Drug Administration has the sole and final authorization to approve the use of irradiated foods for human consumption. At present irradiation of fresh potatoes to prevent sprouting, thus keeping the potatoes fresh for more than a year, and irradiation of wheat and wheat flour to eliminate infestation by insects, are approved by the Food and Drug Administration. (The first irradiated food which won approval was radiation-sterilized bacon, but subsequently the approval was withdrawn.) The radiation-sterilization of several food packaging materials is also permitted.

Food technologists, after having studied food irradiation for over two decades, generally agree that complete radiation-sterilization of food is not feasible at the present. Its costs are prohibitive, and the high doses employed, which destroy the microorganisms and the putrefying enzymes, adversely affect the taste of many foodstuffs. However, research to find solutions to these problems is continuing in most countries.

FOOD POISONING

Acute disturbance or ailment of variable severity following the consumption of food or drink contaminated by bacteria, bacterial toxin, fungi and other parasites, or chemical substances. Formerly it was believed that digesting certain foods created the poisons which caused illnesses, and these illnesses were diagnosed as "ptomaine poisoning" (fr. Gk. *ptōma* carcass). However, it was later discovered that ptomaines, organic substances in decayed food matter, do not cause diseases.

The most frequent bacterial food poisoning is caused by various microorganisms of the genus *Salmonella* (family *Enterobacteriaceae*). The symptoms vary from occasional diarrhea, milder abdominal cramps, and nausea to violent gastrointestinal disturbances marked by severe diarrhea, vomiting, chills, and muscle pain. The most serious salmonella infection is typhoid fever which, especially if untreated, may cause complications resulting in death. Dysentery, a widespread gastrointestinal disorder affecting mainly the densely populated warmer regions of the world, is caused by the consumption of food and drink contaminated with various bacteria of the genus *Shigella* (family *Enterobacteriaceae*), or with various species of amoeba (especially *Endamoeba histolytica*). Dysentery is marked by inflammation of the intestine, frequent diarrhea (the stool sometimes containing blood and mucus), cramps and fever. However, dysentery may subside spontaneously. Bacterial and amoebic food contamination is generally due to poor sanitary environmental conditions, and ingestion of such food is rarely fatal. There are various effective medicines for the treatment of bacterial and amoebic food poisoning, and vaccine against typhoid fever is also available.

In a type of food poisoning which is not caused

directly by bacteria but by the poisonous substance (toxin) produced by them, the bacteria (e.g., *Staphilococcus*) are usually transmitted to the food by infected persons (a pastry cook having a skin infection). Sometimes food handlers or packers may be "carriers," that is, individuals who harbor and transmit the disease-causing organisms without being affected by them. Most often processed meat and fish, creamy pastry, and custards are contaminated, but usually this type of food poisoning is not serious and is of short duration (symptoms may include vomiting, mild diarrhea, and occasionally a temperature).

The most serious but relatively rare food poison botulism, caused by the toxin of the bacillus *Clostridius botulinum*, is nearly always traced to canned and preserved food. The pure toxin is so potent that less than 1/100,000 of a gram can kill a mouse. Insufficient cleaning and improper and faulty preservation processing permit the bacillus to enter the packaged, bottled, or canned food where the low-oxygen environment is favorable to the development of its toxin. The poison affects the nervous system causing double vision, speech disturbances, difficulty in swallowing, dizziness, labored breathing, and ultimately complete respiratory collapse leading to death. (Mortality rate is about 65 percent.) If antitoxin is administered before the development of the serious symptoms, the chances for recovery are good.

Nonbacterial food poisoning may occur after the

consumption of food both of animal and plant origin containing naturally occurring poisonous substances (in certain fish and mushrooms, in fava bean and chick pea), or when the foodstuff contains acquired and accumulated deleterious substances (chemical pesticides on poorly cleaned vegetables, or chemicals such as mercury consumed by animals). Food poisoning, even in its mildest form, may have serious consequences, particularly for people who are afflicted with other ailments or are especially susceptible to certain substances. Therefore, early diagnosis and treatment by a physician is always advisable.

FOOD SUPPLEMENTS

Natural

All vitamins, proteins, minerals, and other food supplements, and some paramedical preparations (e.g., digestion regulator) extracted from natural sources (i.e., plants and animals) without exposure to, and free of, chemicals or other harmful additives, and processed without removing the vital nutrients. See: Subentry on *Synthetic Vitamins* under Vitamins, Health Food Preparations.

Organic

All vitamins, minerals, proteins, and other food supplements which are made, either partially or entirely, by chemical synthesis from organic substances, but not obtained from natural sources. For instance, by legal definition, coal-tar vitamins, or iron compounds made from earth iron and an organic acid, may be labeled "organic." However, such products may not be labeled as "natural" since they are not made from animal or plant sources. See: Subentry on *Synthetic Vitamins* under **Vitamins, Health Food Preparations.**

FROZEN FOODS

The freezing of fresh foods for the purpose of preservation has been a common practice since ancient times among people living in cold climates, especially in the arctic regions and on high mountains. Fresh caught fish, or the whole or cut up carcass of animals were either simply thrown on the ice, buried in ice and snow, or hung up on high poles or on the outside walls of the abodes. Weather-frozen fish have been traded in many countries, and they have been a trade staple in the Great Lakes region since the middle of the last century. Later, various cooling methods were used in freezing meat, fish, and poultry. The advent of mechanical refrigeration greatly enhanced the cold-preservation of practically every food and prompted the development of the frozen food industry. Clarence Birdseye, an American inventor (1886–1956), is credited with the development of the first workable quick-freezing process for preserving food.

Freezing inhibits the growth and action of spoilage-causing microorganisms and arrests enzymatic processes. It does not significantly affect the taste and appearance of the food. After thawing, however, deterioration is rapid, and prolonged thawing results in high nutritional losses. Defrosted food should not be refrozen but prepared and consumed as soon as possible. Frozen foods, if processed properly and kept at the required temperature, have practically all the nutritional values of fresh foods. Some frozen foods, especially vegetables and fruits, contain sometimes added sugar, salt, or some preservatives. Frozen foods cannot be stored at home, unless the refrigerator has a freezer compartment. In the ice cube compartment the temperature is usually not low enough for storing frozen foods for a long period of time. For instance, at zero degree temperature the vitamin content of frozen foods will not be affected, but at 10 degrees and above, there will be a considerable loss in vitamins.

FRUIT

The collective name for a great variety of edible plant products, some of which are called vegetables (tomato, eggplant), or nuts (hazelnut, chestnut). Fruits are a plant's matured ovaries and contain its seeds. In common usage, only those plant products which have soft and pulpy flesh are called fruits (disregarding their different botanical classifications).

Fruits were among the first foods of prehistoric man. Fruit bearing plants cultivated today are the descendants of wild plants, and through domestication and breeding many varieties of the same fruits have been developed. Fruits (and vegetables) are the best source, often the only source, of many vitamins. Fruits contain vitamin A, B_1, B_2, niacin, choline, inositol, folic acid in varying degrees, and they are especially high in vitamin C and the bioflavonoids. Many minerals are present in fruits (iron, copper, phosphorus, sulphur) in different amounts, as well as easily assimilated simple sugars, enzymes, and fruit acids. Since fruits are eaten mostly raw, they tend to be a generally better source of the water-soluble vitamins than vegetables which are usually cooked and cooking easily destroys these vitamins. Fruits are a low-calorie food, though some have a relatively high sugar content (e.g., dates) and these are not recommended in weight-reducing diets. Regular consumption of fresh fruits is necessary for good health and is recommended by all nutritionists.

GINSENG (fr. Ch. *jin-tsan* life of man, root of life)
A perennial herb (*Panax ginseng*) having five-foliolate leaves, bright red berries and an aromatic root. It is widely distributed in the Far Eastern countries. The *Panax quinquefolia,* a similar herb of the ginseng family, is found in North America.

The ginseng root is highly valued in the Orient and is used in the preparation of medicinal drinks, alone or mixed with other herbs, and as a blender for tea. It is supposed to have some calming effect. Ginseng root of the American variety, and pulverized ginseng, alone or mixed with other herbs as a tea preparation, are available in health food stores and in oriental groceries.

GRAHAM FLOUR
A whole wheat flour, named for Sylvester Graham (1794–1851), an American reformer and New England Presbyterian minister who advocated vegetarianism, abstinence from liquor, coffee, and tea. He denounced the use for breadmaking of flours that were finely ground and bolted, and from which the bran and germ were removed. Instead, he recommended the exclusive use of coarsely

ground whole wheat flour. (The graham cracker made from such flour is named for him.) True whole wheat or graham flour must contain the unbolted whole grain. Since the germ contains oil which becomes quickly rancid when exposed to air, graham flour deteriorates fast and cannot be stored for any long period of time. Most commercially baked whole wheat breads have added preservatives (antioxidants) to prevent such deterioration.

GRAIN (fr. L. *granum* seed)

The generic name of the dry and closed fruit (fused with the seed) of plants belonging to the Grass family (wheat, rice, corn). This name is also applied to other plants bearing such fruits (e.g., buckwheat). Most of the important staple grains were first cultivated sometimes between 6000 and 4500 B.C., and became the principal staple of man and his domesticated animals. In primitive agricultural societies everywhere, many magical and religious rites were associated with grains (e.g., rebirth of the vegetation; fertility of man and soil). Several of these beliefs and rites survived, sometimes in a modified form in higher cultures and civilizations. Grain has always been an important produce in commerce and trade among all peoples. The seeds (as grains are commonly called) contain mainly carbohydrates (starch and sugars), but the outer coat (the bran) covering the seed, and the germ of the whole grain, contain several valuable nutrients (vitamins, minerals, proteins).

HEALTH FOOD PREPARATIONS

These are actually complementary foods containing concentrated nutrients derived from one or several sources. Preparations obtained from one source are usually consumed with the ordinary diet. For example, bone meal is mixed into meat dishes such as hamburgers, meat-loafs, stews; skim milk powder into mashed potatoes, soups; sprouts into soups and salads; seaweed powder is used instead of salt and carob powder instead of chocolate. Most preparations containing various nutrients obtained from different sources are blended in a finely ground powder or granules and are to be dissolved in liquids (milk, fruit and vegetable juices, or in plain water). In addition, there are many health food preparations composed of several nutrients and made in a readily edible form such as jelly and candy bars, cookies, and pastes. Health food stores carry a great selection of all types of health food preparations. See: Food Supplements.

HEALTH FOODS

The generic name for all foodstuffs and food supplements which, by virtue of their origin and because of particular methods employed in their cultivation and processing, are considered to be better and more healthful for human nutrition. See: Natural Foods, Organic Foods, Whole Foods.

HERBS

Any of the numerous seed-producing annual, biennial or perennial leafy plants that have no woody stems and die at the end of the growing season. The name "herb" is commonly applied to all plants and their products (seeds, roots, stems, leaves, flowers, and fruits) that are used either for their medicinal properties or for their savory and aromatic qualities as condiments and seasonings in cooking and baking, or as natural food additives. The use of herbs as medicine, brewed into beverages, mixed into foods, chewed or eaten raw, or applied on the skin goes back to the earliest history of mankind. Some of the curative, aphrodisiac, and other extraordinary effects attributed to herbs were based on faulty observations and superstitions. For a long time herbs served as the only sources of medicines. For instance, several species of the fig-wort plants were used medicinally, and one of them, the foxglove (*Digitalis pupurea*) later became an important source of the drug digitalis, a powerful heart stimulant. Herbs were also the chief sources of poisons. The physiologically active principles in herbs are the alkaloids (organic compounds). Most of them are poisons but are, in the proper dosage, therapeutically highly effective. For instance, a drink made from the poison hemlock plant (*Conium maculatum*) was used in executions in Greece and other Mediterranean countries but the same alkaloid (coniine) is now synthetized and used as a sedative and antispasmodic remedy. The advent of chemical synthesis, capable of producing the same active principles uniformly and under controlled conditions, eliminated the direct use and application of herbs as medicinal agents. However, plants still retain their importance as raw material for the manufacture of medicines. There are many advocates of a great variety of herb teas that are reputed to alleviate, and even cure, a variety of diseases ranging from asthma to whooping cough. Homemade herb teas may contain some minute amounts of the active principles, but their therapeutic effectiveness is negligible. As natural condiments and seasoning agents, herbs have a great commercial value. See: **Herb Teas, Spices, Flavoring Agents.**

HERB TEAS

The commonly used name for all beverages brewed from any part of a plant—from the seeds, bulbs, roots, stems, leaves, flowers, and fruits. Herb teas have been popular since antiquity among all peoples, especially as remedies for the cure and prevention of ailments and diseases, and also as "magical" drinks for attaining a certain physical or mental state. Since herb teas usually contain relatively small amounts of herbs and are usually prepared with boiling water, the active principles which have medicinal properties lose their effectiveness or are destroyed. Therefore, most herb teas have a very mild, and in many cases insignificant effect. In order to achieve the claimed results, very great quantities would have to be ingested. There are hundreds of varieties of herb teas, most having several medicinal properties claimed for them. Such claims may vary from country to country, or even from one advocate to the other.

The best known and most commonly used herb teas and some of the beneficial effects they are supposed to have are: aniseed (expels intestinal gases, alleviates nervous headache); balm (relieves indigestion, reduces fever); camomile (alleviates headache, relieves spasm and upset stomach); catnip (expels intestinal gases, relieves headache, produces perspiration); basil (relieves indigestion); dandelion (increases the flow of urine; brew made from the roasted roots is beneficial in rheumatism); elderblossom ("purifies" blood); fennel (stimulates, aids digestion); ground ivy (heals tissues, increases the flow of urine); marjoram (alleviates nervous headache, stimulates, promotes menstruation); mint (stimulates, helps in digestive disorders); nettle (beneficial in rheumatism); rosemary (promotes tissue healing, produces perspiration); sage (stimulates, relieves headache pain and digestive disturbances); thyme (relieves spasm). These and many other herb teas are available in health food stores and in specialty shops. See: Herbs.

HOMINY (of Algonquian Indian origin, probably fr. *minne* grain)

A cereal dish, especially popular in the South. It is made from the broken kernels of corn after the bran (hull) and the germ have been removed. It is boiled until tender and served as a side dish. Sometimes the kernels are ground into very small pieces (hominy grits), boiled in and eaten with milk, or fried as patties. Samp (fr. Narraganset Indian *nasaump* corn mush) is a coarse type of hominy which sometimes includes broken pieces of the hull. Since both cereals are made from the corn grain without the germ and the bran, they contain very little nutrients and are pure carbohydrate foods.

HOMOGENIZATION (to make homogeneous; fr. Gk. *homos* same and *genos* kind)

A process whereby heated milk is forced through small openings in order to break up the milk fat into minute particles that remain suspended and evenly distributed in the milk. The emulsified fat globules become so small that the cream cannot separate. Homogenized milk has a richer flavor and is easier to digest; it is especially recommended for people who are intolerant to fats.

HONEY

A sweet, viscid liquid produced from the nectar of flowers in the sac of the honeybee (*Apis mellifica*) by enzymes which convert the nectar into readily absorbable simple sugars: fructose and glucose. The fluid is stored in open beeswax cells which are sealed only after the deposited liquid, through evaporation of excess water, reaches the consistency of honey. The nutritional value of honey depends on the environmental and climatic conditions under which the flowers grow, while the flavor and color largely depend upon the flowers from which the nectar is taken. Honey, one of the best natural sources of sugar and a pure energy food, contains about 70–80 percent simple sugar; the rest is composed of minerals, small amounts of the vitamin B complex, and some other trace substances. The darker varieties, especially in the comb, contain higher amounts of vitamins than the commercially clarified honey which is filtered through charcoal. The unprocessed honey is referred to as "natural honey." It must be noted that neither the processed nor the unprocessed honey contains any artificial additives. "Organic honey" is unprocessed and produced by bees which collect the nectar from flowers grown on organic farms only, or from wild plants that have not been sprayed with chemicals. See: **Organic Farming and Gardening.**

HORMONES (fr. Gk. *hormōn* to excite or arouse)
Various chemical substances produced by ductless glands and secreted directly into the body fluids, exerting specific and vital effects on the activities of other organs. The hormone producing glands are the pituitary, thyroid and parathyroid, thymus, adrenals, pancreas, the testes in the male, and the

ovaries in the female. These endocrine, that is, internally secreting glands and the hormones produced by them, play a vital role in most functions of the body and mind: growth, sex characteristics, reproduction, metabolism, mental and physical development, personality and behavior. Since there is an interaction between hormones and certain nutrients, dietary insufficiency may result in disturbances of the hormonal balance. It was suggested several decades ago, in particular by German researchers, that hormones are actually vitamins produced by the body, and vitamins are hormones obtained from outside sources. Both are similar in that they are chemical substances needed in minute quantities only, but are essential to life. Glands are subject to increased or decreased activity that will induce an over or underproduction of certain hormones. Overproduction, however, can usually be controlled by the administration of various drugs, while hormonal deficiency is successfully treated in most cases with synthetically produced hormones.

HYDROGENATION

A process whereby hydrogen is added to the molecule of an unsaturated organic compound, such as vegetable oil. It is employed in the manufacture of shortenings (edible fats used in cooking, frying, and baking). During this process, the basic material, usually a vegetable oil, undergoes certain changes and liquid oil condenses to solid fat which will keep even without refrigeration for a long period of time. However, the nutrients in the oil (e.g., vitamins, minerals) are destroyed. Fat-soluble vitamins, such as the vitamins A, D, K, and especially vitamin E, need protection during digestion and absorption which is provided by the vegetable oil used in cooking and baking. Hydrogenated shortenings, however, do not give this necessary protection to the vitamins, and this lack disturbs their absorption and complete utilization by the body. See also: **Margarine,** and subentry on *Vegetable Oils* under **Fats and Oils.**

JUICES

Fruit

The extracted liquid content of the fleshy part (tissues) of various fruits, usually obtained by exerting pressure on the fruit, thereby crushing the tissues and squeezing out the fluid. All fruit juices contain various vitamins (especially vitamin C and A), minerals (e.g., calcium, phosphorus, magnesium), enzymes, easily absorbed simple sugars, and fruit acids, in different amounts. Fresh fruit juices provide vital nutrients in an easily accessible form and, because of the quickly digested fruit sugars, "instant" energy. The refreshing and invigorating effects of the fruit juices are due to their nutritive values rather than to stimulants such as, for instance, the caffeine and cola extract in coffee and soft drinks. If possible fruit juices should be consumed unstrained because the tissue particles contain cellulose (the main constituent of the cell walls) which is beneficial to intestinal motility and aids in the absorption of nutrients. Commercially processed fruit juices are sometimes fortified with vitamins and minerals, but frequently they contain added sugar or artificial sweetener, preservative and coloring agents. The nutritive value of canned fruit juices is usually reduced (except for the sugar content) because of the destructive high temperature used in canning. It is the consensus of nutritionists that fresh (raw) fruit juices are very healthful and their regular consumption (except when contraindicated by certain conditions) is recommended by nutritionists and physicians alike, especially in the diet of growing children. See: **Cider.**

Vegetable

The liquid content of the tissues of the green leaves (e.g., cabbage), fruits (e.g., tomato), or the roots (e.g., carrot) of various plants, commonly called vegetables. It is usually extracted by grinding the leaves and roots, and then straining the juice, or by crushing the fleshy part without straining, thereby obtaining a thick juice. All vegetable juices contain various vitamins (vitamin A, sev-

eral vitamins of the B-complex, vitamin C), and
minerals (iron, sulphur, magnesium, phosphorus),
enzymes, acids, and salt, in different amounts.
Vegetable juices are generally not as popular as
fruit juices because of their strange and sometimes
bitter taste. However, most commercially processed vegetable juices are mixed and blended to
make them tastier. Some brands contain sugar or
artificial sweetener, preservatives, or other additives. Canned vegetable juices are usually fortified
with vitamin C and other vitamins, and particularly with those which are easily destroyed by the
high temperatures necessary in canning. While,
generally, no exaggerated therapeutic claims are
attached to fruit juices, vegetable juice advocates
assert that regular consumption of various vegetable juices can prevent and cure many disorders
and diseases (turnip juice is useful in the treatment of anemia, liver and kidney disorders; dandelion juice relieves the symptoms of asthma and
helps in circulatory troubles; parsley juice stimulates the nerves and prevents the hardening of the
arteries). All vegetable juices, as with fruit juices,
are healthy and nutritious, but the above claims
have not been substantiated by medical evidence.

LACTOSE

Milk sugar; a carbohydrate occurring only in the
milk of mammals and not found in plants. It is an

important ingredient in the diet of young mammals, including man. As are cane and beet sugar (sucrose), lactose is a double sugar but it is less sweet. (For an explanation of double sugar, see **Sugar.**) Upon fermentation by bacteria in the intestinal tract, lactose yields lactic acid that helps in absorbing the minerals calcium and phosphorus, and promotes the utilization of the vitamins B_2 and B_6. Because of their lactic acid content, sour milk, yogurt, and cottage cheese are easier to digest than plain milk. See: Subentry on *Fermented milk* under **Milk, Yogurt.**

LEAVENING AGENTS (fr. L. *levare* to raise)

Chemical compounds that produce gas bubbles in the dough of bread and other flour foods. Preheating of the dough will expand the bubbles, and the increased heat during baking will change the proteins in the flour, milk, and eggs. The changed proteins, by forming protective shields around the bubbles, will prevent shrinkage or collapse of the baked products upon cooling. Next to the biological leavens (yeast and bacteria), potassium acid tartrate (cream of tartar) has been used for centuries for the same purpose. Later, baking soda (sodium bicarbonate) became the preferred leavening agent for many generations. Today, all leavening agents used by the food industry are chemical substances. Many times these substances are used in combination to achieve the best results, especially in preleavened mixes (e.g., cakes, rolls). Commercial baking powders usually consist of sodium bicarbonate with an acid salt and starch, or of sodium aluminum sulfate with calcium phosphate. These latter substances will retain the gas in the dough, thus permitting the storage (refrigeration) of the dough for later use. The use of artificial leavening agents must be stated on the product's package or label. See: **Additives, Yeast.**

LECITHIN (fr. Gk. *lekithos* egg yolk)

Any of the several colorless, crystalline alcohol-soluble compounds occurring in animal and plant tissues, for example, in the brain, nerves, semen, egg yolk, soybean. It is a combination of fatty acids, especially of the essential unsaturated fatty acids, and is an important source of two B vitamins: choline and inositol. Lecithin metabolizes fats, including cholesterol. It prevents certain types of fatigue and weakness, and is helpful in various skin disorders. It is obtainable only from natural, unprocessed foods like unrefined vegetable oils, eggs, and wheat germ. Extracted from soybean, it is available in health food stores as a food supplement in tasty, granular form or as a spread, or in liquid form in bottles.

LIQUID FOOD

Liquids containing various nutrients such as milk, soups, vegetable and fruit juices are considered "liquid foods." In a stricter sense, however, the term "liquid food," or "liquid meal," applies to commercially processed mixtures, usually containing soybean flour, malt, bone meal, wheat germ, and brewer's yeast, with added proteins, vitamins, and minerals, in skim milk, or similar mixtures in powder form which have to be dissolved in skim milk, vegetable or fruit juices, or in plain water. Such liquid foods are used chiefly in weight-reducing diets as substitutes for a variety of ordinary foods, and in many cases they replace most or all of the ordinary menus. Advocates of the practically fat-free liquid diet claim that it provides all the necessary nutrients, and is a safe and quick way to lose weight. They also recommend staying on the liquid diet in order to prevent obesity. Many nutritionists, however, oppose the exclusive consumption of liquid meals because they do not always contain all the vital nutrients, do not provide enough fat intake (both the saturated and unsaturated fats are important in nutrition), and do not supply the bulk material necessary for proper intestinal metabolism. See: **Bulk Food, Fletcherism, Macrobiotics.**

MACROBIOTICS (fr. Gk. *makros* long, great, and *biōtikos* living, lit. a special way of life)

A particular kind of diet, based on the principles of the cooking and selection of nutriments, as practiced for centuries in Zen Buddhist monasteries. It is also the basis and center of certain beliefs and teachings, involving practically everything from ancient Chinese cosmology and Buddhist philosophy to the prevention and cure of disease. According to its basic philosophy, the universe consists of two opposite principles which are interacting and complementary, the yin and the yang (e.g., masculine and feminine, light and dark, expansion and constriction). The equilibrium between the yin and yang forces, known as the Unique Principle, creates the order of the universe. Since all nutrients, as everything in the world, are either more yin (e.g., tomato, pork, sugar) or more yang (e.g., rice, carrot, egg), the correct macrobiotic diet will balance the yin and yang in man, thus giving him health, vitality, happiness, inner peace, and longevity. All problems are created by the imbalance of yin and yang, and this can be prevented, corrected and eliminated by attaining the yin and yang balance in oneself through the macrobiotic diet and way of life.

Macrobiotic philosophy and diet were "rediscovered" and introduced to Europe in the late forties, and to America in the early sixties, by the late Nyoiti Sakurazawa under his Westernized name, George Ohsawa. The diet consists of ten basic recipes, all containing various amounts of grains and cereals, especially unpolished rice, as the main ingredients. Selected vegetables, sea produce, seeds, and nuts are included according to their yin and yang properties. Fruits are usually avoided, and the least possible amount of animal products is used. All foodstuffs should be natural, unprocessed, and free of any artificial additives. Liquid intake should not exceed eight ounces per day but all solid food should be chewed at least 50 times until it becomes liquid. According to advocates, macrobiotic philosophy can be absorbed faster, and a higher standard of health can be achieved sooner if food is chewed 100 to 150 times. In preparing macrobiotic food, as well as eating it, various rituals are observed.

A variety of macrobiotic foodstuffs are prepared and available in packages and jars, for example, Miso, a paste made from soybean, wheat, and sea salt; Shoyu sauce, also made from soybean, wheat, and sea salt, and fermented for several years; Kokoh, a mixture of roasted rice, soybean, sesame seed, and oatmeal, eaten cooked with milk; Gomasio, roasted and ground sesame seeds with sea salt, used as a seasoning powder; Mu tea, a mixture of ginseng and some fifteen other herbs; Lotus tea, made from the dried roots of the lotus flower. Macrobiotic food is available in specialty shops and restaurants, and in some health food stores. See: **Organic Foods, Fletcherism.**

MALT

Grain, usually barley, which has been steeped in water, softened, germinated, and then dried. It contains the sugars maltose and dextrin, and the enzyme diastase. Malt is used in brewing and distilling alcoholic beverages, such as beer and whiskey. Its high carbohydrate and protein contents make it a nourishing food. It also aids in the digestion of other starchy foods. In medicine, malt extract (or fluid extract) is used sometimes as an adjuvant therapy chiefly to promote gaining weight in wasting diseases (e.g., in tuberculosis, cholera). A powder prepared from malt and dried milk is used to make the popular beverage malted milk.

MARGARINE (F fr. Gk. *margaron* pearl)

A food product, sometimes referred to as "artificial butter" or oleomargarine, made usually from vegetable oils, occasionally in combination with animal fats. It was invented by a French chemist around the middle of the last century, and was first produced mainly from beef fat (oleo). Later other animal fats and vegetable oils were used. Today, over 90 percent of all margarines manufactured in the United States is made from vegetable oils, chiefly corn, soybean, and cottonseed. The extracted oils are refined, deodorized, and churned with cultured or ripened skim milk to the consistency of butter. Salt is added to some brands. Nearly all brands are fortified with vitamins A and D. Margarine is easily digested. It contains almost twice as many unsaturated fatty acids as butter (which is why people who wish to reduce the cholesterol intake in their diet use it as a butter substitute), but it yields the same number of calories. Some brands of margarine are manufactured with hydrogenated oils. See: **Hydrogenation.**

MEAT

In general, the flesh of all animals used as food; in particular, the flesh of mammals (cattle, swine, sheep, and game animals) as distinct from fish and fowl (poultry and game fowl). It has not been determined when man became a meat eater, but it is known that meat has been his staple food since prehistoric times. Meat consumption depended on local availability, as it still does to a certain degree.

Meat has always been the principal food of people living in the arctic regions, or on high mountains where vegetation is scanty or nonexistent. The first meat probably eaten was the raw flesh of animals found dead. As man developed his tools, animals were hunted and trapped. Later, experience taught man that frying and cooking the meat, especially in warmer regions, prevented spoilage and the diseases caused by eating contaminated raw flesh.

Meat is composed chiefly of water, fat, and proteins containing all the essential amino acids. It also supplies various minerals and vitamins—these are especially abundant in the organ meats. Because of its very high nutritional value, meat is considered an important and necessary part of the daily diet. Under ordinary conditions, meat is easily and completely digested. Raw meat requires about two hours' digestion, while well-done meat is digested in about four hours. The fatter the meat, the longer the digestive process. Almost all the proteins and over 95 percent of the fat are utilized by the body. While sugar and starchy foods are digested faster, only 75 to 85 percent of the proteins in vegetables, fruits, and cereals are assimilated and used by the body.

The raising of animals for food, as well as the processing of meat (slaughtering, preparation of the carcasses, packaging, distribution) are regulated by federal and state laws. Meats (including fish and fowl) sold to the public must be government inspected. If so desired by the processor, meat may be graded according to a classification set by the Department of Agriculture; this grade, however, does not necessarily determine the nutritional value of a special cut. The grading usually classifies the meat into prime, choice, good, medium, common, and low cuts. Good meat may be recognized by a firm texture evenly interspersed with fat, a clear and uniform color (which does not have to be always "deep red"), little moisture, and clean odor. The so-called high-grade meats are not richer in proteins and other nutrients than the low-grade meats which are especially suitable for stews, meat loafs, and soups. Pork liver, for instance, regarded by many people as the least desirable and, therefore, the cheapest of all livers, is richer in nutrients, particularly in iron, complete proteins, and vitamin A than the more expensive beef and calf liver. The "hanging" of meat for a certain period allows the accelerated formation of lactic acid in the muscular walls and connective tissues which soften the meat. Vinegar or a meat tenderizer (a commercial enzyme preparation) can be used for the same purpose. A slight greyish discoloration of the surface of the meat is due to exposure to the air and does not mean it is inferior in quality. Although meat has always been universally recognized as one of the most important foods essential for maintaining good health, it has nevertheless been subject to prohibitions and prejudices either because of dietary theories or religious beliefs. See: **Meat Tenderizer.**

MEAT TENDERIZER

A colorless, crystalline powder containing the protein splitting enzyme (papain) of the unripe papaya fruit. When applied to raw meat before cooking, the powder is absorbed into the connective tissues of the meat and will render it soft by breaking down ("predigesting") the proteins. The meat tenderizer is a natural product and contains no chemicals. It is sold in most grocery stores.

METABOLISM (fr. Gk. *metaballein* to change)

The sum of all physical and chemical processes involved in the sustenance of life, especially the building up of cells through assimilation of food, the repair of the tissues (anabolism), the transformation of food into energy for vital processes, and the destruction and elimination of waste from the body (catabolism).

MILK

Regular

A fluid, secreted by the mammary glands of the breasts or the udders of female animals (mammals) that suckle their young. It is a nearly complete food for infants and a highly nutritious complementary food for adults. It is composed of fat (butterfat), suspended in a solution containing proteins, milk sugar (lactose), calcium, phosphorus, and other minerals, and enzymes. It is a major source of the vitamins A and B_2 (riboflavin), and also contains the vitamins C and E. The vitamin D content of milk is usually supplemented with added vitamin D, or it is fortified by ultraviolet irradiation. Sometimes irradiated yeast is mixed into the fodder of the cows in order to increase the vitamin D content of the milk.

Milk and milk products (e.g., butter) were already important parts of the diet many thousands of years ago, and the milk obtained from many different animals (cow, goat, ewe, mare, yak, buffalo, llama, reindeer) was used as food in various parts of the world. Today, however, 90 percent of the milk consumed in one form or another in the world is obtained from cows. In most countries milk is pasteurized for human consumption, and in many it is also homogenized. Pasteurization destroys various nutrients in the milk and thus reduces its nutritional value but it checks bacterial growth, making it safer to drink and increasing keeping qualities. It does this without boiling, which destroys practically all nutrients.

When the fat content of milk is removed, the remainder is called *skim* milk which is usually drunk in weight-reducing diets. Although most of the vitamin A is removed with the cream, skim milk is still rich in other valuable nutrients. *Concentrated* or *evaporated* milk is produced by partial evaporation of the water content, and when sugar is added, it is called *condensed* milk. Both forms retain the nutrients. *Powdered* or dried milk is manufactured by evaporation of the water content. After complete evaporation of the water, the dried granules of the milk are recovered. Powdered milk is an exceptionally rich and concentrated source of all milk nutrients. As a supplement (added to soups and gravies, mixed into meatloafs, hamburgers) it will contribute considerably to the supply of necessary nutrient. See: **Butter, Cheese.**

Buttermilk

The liquid residue left after churning cream into butter. It is rich in water-soluble minerals, and contains proteins, vitamin B_2, and various enzymes. It has a pleasant and refreshing but slightly sour taste due to its lactic acid content. It is easily digested. Buttermilk is practically fat-free and, therefore, it is very low in calories. It is a healthy, nutritious beverage and is especially recommended in weight-reducing diets. Buttermilk derived from butter made from certified raw milk is available in health food stores.

Certified Raw Milk

The use of ordinary raw milk was always considered as a possible danger to human health. Often the cows had infectious diseases (e.g., tuberculosis) that went unnoticed because of negligent supervision and poor or nonexistent medical care of the animals. The unsanitary conditions under which cows were kept, fed, and milked often caused severe contamination of the milk. These facts led to the enactment of the pasteurization laws in most countries. However, it soon became apparent that pasteurization, while it inactivates many of the disease-causing microorganisms, also reduces the milk's nutritional value and destroys the phosphatase enzymes which are necessary for the absorption of the minerals (calcium and phosphorus).

Health inspection of cows producing milk destined to be pasteurized is infrequent because it is assumed that pasteurization will eliminate any contamination. At the end of the last century, a New Jersey physician, Dr. Henry L. Coit, conceived the idea of "certified raw milk" and organized the first Medical Milk Commission. Safety regulations were laid down for the production of raw milk for direct consumption. Today, the production and distribution of certified raw milk is regulated by state and county laws. The cows must receive daily veterinarian inspection, are shampooed daily, and milked by sterilized machines. The workers employed by the certified raw milk industry must also undergo medical examinations at regular intervals. The cows are fed a balanced diet year round. Their milk is constantly tested in laboratories both for quantity and types of micro-organisms. *Certified* means that the milk was produced in strict compliance with the rules governing every phase of the production. Certified raw milk is highly nutritious and has an excellent taste. It is not homogenized, and if left to sit the cream will separate. Certified raw milk should be consumed as soon as possible after production. Under refrigeration, however, it will usually remain fresh for several days. Certified raw milk and products made from it (sour milk, cottage cheese, cheeses) are available in health food stores.

Fermented Milk

A food product made of whole or skimmed milk curdled to a semiliquid state by fermentation with any of the several lactic acid producing micro-organisms of the family *Lactobacteriaceae*. Various types of fermented milk of cow, goat, sheep, horse, camel, and llama have been produced for centuries by herdsmen in Asia, Eastern and Southern Europe, Scandinavia, Africa, and South America: the koumiss, an effervescent alcohol-containing beverage made by the Mongols and Tartars from yeast fermented mare's milk; the kefir (kefyr), made in the regions of the Caucasus from cow's or mare's milk by fermenting it with kefir grains; the kaeldermaelk, a viscous, ropy fermented milk food of Scandinavia. The best known and most popular fermented milk products are sour milk and yogurt. (Sour milk is sometimes mistaken for buttermilk which is not fermented but is a by-product left after churning butter from cream.) Sour milk is easier to digest than plain sweet milk and, because of its high lactic acid content, it enhances the absorption of the minerals in the milk and retards the growth of putrefactive organisms in the intestinal tract. Sour milk, made from certified raw milk is available in health food stores. See: **Yogurt.**

Goat's Milk

It is widely used in the countries of the Middle East and the Mediterranean regions as part of the daily diet, either in liquid form or made into cheese, or as an additive in cooking and baking. Fresh goat's milk has a specific rich, creamy flavor. As far as nutritional values are concerned, there is no significant difference between goat's and cow's milk. Because goat's milk is naturally homogenized, as is human milk, it is more easily digested than cow's milk. It is sometimes recommended for infants and children who are allergic or sensitive to cow's milk, or for persons who are generally intolerant to fats. In health food stores, certified raw goat milk and cheeses made of it are available. Goat's milk is also sold in dried powder form.

MILLET

The common name for any of the numerous varieties of an annual, small-seeded cereal plant (especially *Panicum miliaceum*) of the Grass family, grown and cultivated since ancient times for its grain. (The sowing of millet became part of religious ceremonies in China more than 4,500 years ago.) In most parts of Asia, especially in China and India, and in Africa, as well as in many countries in Europe, millet is used as food, both for men and animals. In China and India, millet is ground to flour for breadmaking. In the United States it is cultivated mainly for forage and hay, and the grains are used for feeding poultry and pet birds. The grains of millet are rich in lecithin, proteins, and calcium. It is only recently that millet became more popular as a breakfast cereal in America. It can also be used in baking. Millet is available in health food stores in unprocessed form (it cooks quickly), and in processed form as a tasty cereal.

MINERALS

General

Inorganic substances having definite physical properties and certain characteristic chemical compositions. Minerals are abundant in nature, some of them are elements (carbon, gold, lead), but most of them are chemical compounds. To a great extent, the human body is composed of various minerals and does require a constant supply of them in order to grow, and function properly. Minerals are vital for the bones, internal organs, nerves, and muscles.

There is an interrelation between minerals and vitamins; without minerals the vitamins cannot be fully utilized. Minerals prevent the blood and tissue fluids from becoming too acid. If acidity of the blood remains constant over a long period of time, serious disorders will result. Minerals contribute to the alkaline reserve and keep the proper balance between the alkaline and acid content of the body. The glandular secretion of hormones is stimulated by minerals. Deficiency in any of the minerals may cause adverse reactions and trigger off grave illnesses.

All foods contain minerals in varying degrees, some of them are in animal products, and others in plants, but some minerals are found in both. There is an all-around interaction between minerals and other nutrients. Inadequate supply of minerals hinders this interaction, thus absorption and utilization of the minerals themselves as well as that of the other nutrients will be incomplete. The average daily diet does not always contain all the minerals in sufficient quantities necessary for good health. The Food and Nutrition Board of the National Research Council established the daily allowances for some of the minerals. While the need for the other minerals has been determined, the minimum daily requirement is not exactly known. Many nutritionists regard the suggested amounts as insufficient and recommend more. Many commercially processed foods contain added minerals. The required minerals, their functions in the body and their food sources as well as the trace minerals (which are effective and required in infinitesimal quantities) are described below.

Calcium

A silver white metallic element which does not occur alone in nature but only in combination, and as such is found widely distributed in various compounds. It is a component of most animal and plant matter. Calcium is the most abundant of all the minerals in the body. It is essential to the formation of the bones and teeth where practically all calcium is stored. Calcium also functions in the regulation of heart rhythm and in blood clotting. It maintains strong bones and prevents rickets and dental decay. It helps to control neuromuscular weakness and irritability. For the proper utilization and assimilation of calcium, a sufficient amount of vitamin D is necessary and, to a lesser degree, the vitamin A and the vitamin B complex. Without phosphorus and iron, the assimilation of calcium is retarded. Growing children, pregnant and nursing women, and the elderly have an especially great need for calcium. Recent research indicates that increased calcium intake may have a beneficial influence on certain cardio-vascular diseases. It has been found that calcium deficiency is nationwide. The richest sources of calcium are milk and milk products. Milk provides an acid medium needed for the best absorption of calcium. In general, vegetables and fruits are poor in calcium. However, kale, broccoli, almonds, and soybean flour are good sources. The National Research Council recommends 0.8 gram as the daily allowance for a healthy adult, and 1.2 to 1.4 grams for a teenager. (One quart of raw milk supplies about one gram of calcium.) Calcium is found in many foods in varying amounts.

Chlorine

A nonmetallic element which does not occur by itself in nature but in a great variety of compounds. (For instance, common salt, sodium chloride, is a compound formed by chlorine with sodium.) It is widely used in water purification; as a disinfectant and antiseptic; in bleaching and fumigating. It is used in medicine in various compounds (e.g., chloroform, an anesthetic agent). Chlorine stimulates the production of digestive juices, such as the hydrochloric acid in the stomach. It aids in maintaining the water balance in the body, and acts as a cleanser in the waste removal processes. Chlorine plays a role also in the distribution of hormones, and in muscle contractions.

The best sources are table salt, raw meat, leafy vegetables, beets, radishes, and ripe olives.

Copper

A malleable metallic element, found mostly in combined forms, though small amounts occur free in nature. It is present in very minute quantities in the animal body and in various plants. Copper is necessary for the utilization of iron to metabolize food into hemoglobin. (Hemoglobin in the blood cells carries the life-supporting oxygen throughout the body.) Formation of the skin pigment depends on copper which also plays a role in the prevention of premature graying of the hair. Copper deficiency causes a certain anemic condition, general weakness, and impaired breathing. It is usually well supplied in a great variety of foods, the best sources being green leafy vegetables, liver, sea food, egg yolk, dried fruits (especially apricots), and whole grains.

Iodine

A nonmetallic element, obtained from salt deposits. It forms several compounds with other non-metallic elements (e.g., phosphorus), hydrogen, and with most metals. Iodine is used in medicine as an antiseptic (tincture), and as a component of various drugs. It is vital to the production of thyroxin, a hormone produced by the thyroid gland. Deficiency of iodine causes goiter, and the underproduction of the thyroid hormone usually results in sluggishness, overweight, poor blood circulation, and impaired mental capacity. Iodine is also important for healthy hair, nails, and complexion. The body contains about 25 milligrams of iodine, of which more than two thirds is concentrated in the thyroid gland. The rest is in the tissues and blood, and in the other endocrine glands, especially in the ovaries. It is a trace mineral, that is, only a very minute quantity is required of it. All sea foods, both animal and vegetable, are rich sources of iodine. Land animals and plants also contain iodine but the amount of it varies because it depends on the iodine's presence in the soil from which the plants absorb. Codfish, cod liver oil, haddock, oysters, sardines, and seaweed have a high iodine content. Garlic, spinach, cabbage, and onion are also good sources. The iodine content of the plants varies with the seasons, and it is usually higher in the autumn and winter. Iodine in food form is nontoxic, and the body eliminates the unused iodine. Therefore, many nutritionists advocate a greater intake of iodine than the estimated amount needed in order to prevent a possible deficiency. The suggested daily requirement is probably one microgram per kilogram (2.2 pounds of body weight. (One pound of sardines contains 164 microgram of iodine; one pound of oranges has one microgram of iodine.)

Iron

A silver white, magnetic, malleable element which rarely occurs uncombined in nature (except in meteorites). It is the fourth most abundant element comprising approximately 5 percent of the earth's crust, and it is vital to biological processes in most animals and many plants. Iron is essential to the formation of hemoglobin which carries oxygen in the red blood cells to all the cells in the body, and removes the body's waste product, carbon dioxide. Without oxygen the cells would die.

Iron is also important in the metabolism of various other nutrients. Iron deficiency causes anemia (fr. Gk. *anaimia* lit. bloodlessness), though not all forms of anemia are caused by this. Anemic conditions are characterized by constant fatigue, tired, pale skin, and low resistance to infectious diseases. Severe anemia can cause mental disorders and heart failure. Generally, anemia is more prevalent in women than men. It is estimated that about 90 percent of all women in America have hemoglobin deficiency in varying degrees. The national average of the blood's hemoglobin content is about 15 to 30 percent below normal.

The best food sources of iron are the organ meats, especially pork and beef liver, egg yolk, oysters, wheat germ, peanut, soybean, apricots, and barley. Pernicious anemia, the most severe form of anemia, is now successfully treated with vitamin B_{12}. The National Research Council recommends a minimum daily intake of 10 milligrams of iron for a man, and 18 milligrams for a woman and teenage girls and boys. During pregnancy and lactation, and if the menstrual flow is excessive, the daily intake should be increased. (Two ounces of pork liver supply about 15 milligrams of iron.)

Magnesium

A silver white malleable metallic element which is abundant in nature and is found in a great variety of compounds. In the form of salts, it is used as food by plants, and it is one of the constituents of the green pigment (chlorophyll) in the plants. In the body, about 70 percent of the magnesium is deposited in the bones and, as are calcium and phosphorus, it is important in the growth and maintenance of healthy bones and teeth. Magnesium is necessary for the proper utilization of vitamin C, for normal muscle and heart activity, and is believed to play a role as a coenzyme (by activating other enzymes) in fat metabolism and in the building of proteins. Magnesium deficiency may cause degenerative diseases of the bones and teeth, great neuromuscular irritability, and adverse effects on the blood pressure. In experimental clinical studies, magnesium (in the form of magnesium sulphate) has been found to reduce high blood cholesterol levels, and to dissolve or to prevent the formation of kidney and gall stones. Some magnesium compounds are important in medicine and have been used as therapeutic agents for a long time (e.g., milk of magnesia, Epsom salt). In the daily diet the best sources of magnesium are green vegetables, whole grains, and nuts. The daily adult requirement has been estimated at 250–300 milligrams.

Manganese

A metallic element, harder than iron; it does not occur by itself in nature but is found widely distributed in various compounds. Manganese is important in the proper functioning of the glands (most of it is concentrated in the liver, pancreas, and adrenal glands). It is necessary for reproduction, and it promotes milk formation in the female. (Eggs of hens fed on manganese-free diet do not hatch, and female animals deficient in manganese lack any maternal instinct.) Manganese is also interrelated with the metabolism of vitamins B_1 and E. Best sources are leafy green vegetables, whole grains, beans, bananas, liver, egg yolk, and nuts.

Phosphorus

A nonmetallic element which does not occur alone in nature but is found in combination with other minerals. It is present in the tissues of animals and plants. Phosphorus acts as an hardening agent in the bones and teeth; it is important for brain functions, and for muscle and nerve activity. Phosphorus deficiency results in rickets, brittle bones and teeth, loss of appetite, general weakness, and retarded growth. Phosphorus is as vital to the body as calcium is. Without adequate amounts of calcium, however, phosphorus cannot be absorbed and properly utilized. Phosphorus and calcium are assimilated only when vitamin D is present. The best sources of phosphorus are the protein and calcium-rich foods, that is, meat, poultry, eggs, cheese, milk, nuts, and soybean. Sufficient consumption of protein foods usually provides the necessary quantity of phosphorus. The daily intake for adults should be approximately one and a half times that of calcium or about 16 milligrams. Because of widespread calcium deficiency, many nutritionists recommend additional intake of calcium in order to ensure the proper assimilation of phosphorus.

Potassium

A silver white, soft, metallic element found abundantly in nature combined with other minerals, and in animal and plant tissues. Various potassium salts are used therapeutically in medicine (e.g., potassium bromide, a sedative and antispasmodic), as antiseptics and disinfectants (e.g., potassium permanganate), and as antidotes for certain poisons (e.g., potassium iodide). It is an important mineral, especially during the years of rapid growth. It aids in the disposal of the body's waste products, in the proper functioning of the nervous and cardio-vascular systems and, together with phosphorus, promotes the transportation of oxygen to the brain cells. Children need more potassium than adults. Potassium deficiency may lead to growth retardation and faulty bone development. Lack of potassium can cause nervous ailments, loss of mental agility, and kidney damage. Under normal circumstances, however, potassium deficiency is rare. Whole grains, dried legumes such as beans, peas, and lentils, potatoes, figs, leafy green vegetables, fish, and meat are all good sources of potassium. The estimated daily requirement is about 0.8 to 1.5 grams.

Sodium

A silver white metallic element, not found alone in nature, but widely distributed in compounds. The various compounds are commercially very important and are utilized in nearly every industry. In medicine, sodium compounds have long been used and they constitute the main ingredients in a great variety of pharmaceutical preparations. The common salt (sodium chloride) is a compound formed by sodium with chlorine. It is the most directly used mineral and is an extremely important constituent of the diet of man and animals. Salt is a life-sustaining mineral. Under normal circumstances the healthy body requires a regular daily intake of at least ten grams of salt. Nearly all foods contain salt to varying degrees. See: Salt.

Sulphur

A nonmetallic element which appears in many forms and is widely distributed in nature, either free or in various compounds. It is used in the manufacture of disinfectants, pesticides, bleaching agents, matches, rubber, and paper. Sulphur is the basic constituent of the sulfa drugs. Sulphur is a component of certain amino acids in proteins. It is needed for healthy skin, hair, and nails. It promotes the metabolism of other minerals by the liver, and aids in the secretion of bile. With sulphur deficiency the ingestion of inorganic sulphur in any form (as a supplement) will not help since only the sulphur-containing amino acids of proteins can be utilized by the body. The best sources are the protein foods, and cabbage, brussels sprouts, wheat germ, and lentil. The estimated minimum daily requirement is more than one gram.

Zinc

A bluish white metallic element occurring abundantly in nature in various compounds. These compounds are widely used in the chemical, pharmaceutical and cosmetic industries, and the metal itself is of great commercial importance. Zinc is essential to the growth and development of animals and plants. In the human body, most of it is concentrated in the thyroid glands, but it is present in all tissues. It is a constituent of insulin (a hormone secreted by the pancreas), and because of its interrelation with vitamin B_1, it aids the metabolism of carbohydrates and proteins. It is reported that zinc is probably necessary for the production of the male hormone and thus it may influence healthy reproductive functions. In leukemia and diabetic conditions the zinc content of the body is decreased. It is, however, not known whether this is caused by the diseases or whether the low zinc content is a contributing factor to the rise of these conditions. The symptoms of zinc deficiency resemble those of vitamin B_1 deficiency. The best food sources for zinc have not been clearly determined, though organ meats, legumes (beans, lentils and so on) are recommended. It is estimated that the minimum daily requirement is about ten milligrams.

In addition to copper, iodine, and manganese, there are other *trace minerals* which are found in the tissues, glands, and body fluids in infinitesimal quantities. These trace minerals are *boron, bromine, cobalt, fluorine, nickel,* and *silver*. They influence the growth, the reproductive functions, cellular health, and mental activity. The average normal diet provides these trace minerals, and specific deficiency cases in these minerals are rare.

MOLASSES (fr. L. *mellaceus* honeylike)
The residue left after the crystallization of sugar, a thick, sweet, viscid syrup having a light to dark brown color and a distinctive strong taste. The blackstrap molasses, or sugarhouse molasses, ob-

tained in the process of sugar refining, contains a relatively high amount of iron and, to a lesser degree, some other minerals, and vitamins of the B complex (except B_1 and folic acid). The dark variety has more nutritional value (about fifteen times more iron) and less sugar than the lighter variety. Molasses is used mostly as a food supplement, sometimes in nutritional anemia, and as a general sweetening agent in cooking and baking. Claims that molasses has a direct therapeutic effect on certain ailments as well as other medicinal properties have not been proven. Health food stores carry various brands of bottled molasses.

MUSHROOMS

Any of the several edible, nonpoisonous fungi, especially the common meadow mushroom (*Agraricus campestris*), typically having a fleshy body which consists of a stem bearing a dome-shaped cap. Fresh mushrooms are rich in folic acid and contain several other vitamins of the B complex. They are the only known nonanimal source of vitamin D. In America, mushrooms are generally used as a flavoring as in soups and gravies, while in Europe they are also eaten as vegetables. Another fleshy, edible globular fungus, the truffle (genus *Tuber*) grows below the ground's surface in several southern European countries. Eaten alone, cooked or fried, or added as flavoring to other foods, it is considered a delicacy. Truffles have not been successfully cultivated and are usually hunted with dogs and hogs which can smell them below the ground. Mushrooms and truffles are available fresh or in cans, jars, or dried in packages.

NATURAL FOODS

All foodstuffs of plant or animal origin which are processed without the removal of the natural nutrients, and are free of chemical additives (e.g., preservatives, flavoring and coloring agents, and synthetic supplements). In most cases, the removed nutrients (e.g., proteins, vitamins, and minerals) cannot always be substituted completely, or even sufficiently, by synthetic nutrients. Natural foods are synonymous with "whole foods." See: Whole Foods, Organic Foods, Health Foods.

NUTRIENT (fr. L. *nutrire* to suckle, to nourish)

An important substance or ingredient in food that affects the metabolic processes and provides nourishment for the body (e.g., a vitamin).

NUTRIMENT (fr. L. *nutrimentum* nourishment)

Materials, specifically food and drink that contain the necessary ingredients to nourish or promote growth and to repair the natural wastage of organic life, thereby maintaining the life of the organism that ingests them.

NUTRITION

The food materials that nourish, and the processes that utilize these materials by separating and absorbing them for maintenance, growth, repair, reproduction, and general sustenance of the body.

NUTRITIONAL THERAPY

The use of a special diet in the treatment of an ailment or disease due chiefly to nutritional deficiency (e.g., in anemic conditions the daily intake of iron-rich foods, such as liver and other organ meats, apricots, parsley, and whole wheat products); or a particular diet for the purpose of gaining or reducing weight. Generally, in nutritional therapy drugs (chemicals) are not used, and the prescribed special diet must be followed for a longer period of time. Sometimes, however, nutritional therapy is employed in the correction of an acute condition not necessarily caused by nutritional deficiency (e.g., grated apple as an exclusive diet for infants in the treatment of diarrheal conditions). See: **Diet.**

NUTS

The common name for a great variety of edible seeds, or of fruits which have edible kernels, enclosed in hard or brittle shells. Botanically, nuts are one-seeded fruits, as the true nuts like hazelnut, chestnut, and acorn. The most popular "nuts" are actually not true nuts, for example, the coconut, pecan nut, and walnut are fruits; the pistachio, Brazil nut, and cashew are seeds; and the peanut is a legume. Nuts belong to the oldest foods of mankind. They were originally gathered from wild trees, but now many nut-bearing trees and shrubs are cultivated commercially. In many parts of the world, especially in tropical and subtropical countries, nuts constitute a staple food. In the United States nuts are used mostly in confectionery, as seasonings, or as snacks. Various nuts (e.g., coconut, almonds, peanuts) also provide valuable raw materials for the food, chemical, cosmetic and other industries.

Nuts are highly nutritious, and for their size they contain about twice the amount of nutrients supplied by any other foodstuff, save seeds. They are a good source of proteins, although the proteins are biologically not as effective as those of animal origin. All nuts are rich in oil, having a high content of unsaturated fatty acids. Nuts contain vitamin E, several vitamins of the B complex, and various minerals. Organically grown nuts, dried, roasted, salted, and unsalted, and food products made from nuts (e.g., peanut butter, almond paste and milk, coconut milk) are available in most health food stores. Many nutritionists recommend the regular consumption of nuts as a snack instead of the more commonly eaten sweet and starchy foods. See: **Peanut, Organic Peanut Butter, Seeds.**

OAT

A widely cultivated annual cereal (grain) plant (*Avena sativa*) of the Grass family. The domestication of oat began relatively late (perhaps around 2,500 B.C.) as compared to that of wheat which was grown in Egypt almost seven thousand years ago. A moist and temperate climate is favorable to growing oat, and its cultivation in northern Europe was widespread when the horse was first used by man. From northern Europe, oat was introduced to the Mediterranean regions and other parts of the world. Today, the leading oat producing countries are the United States, the USSR, Canada, and northern Europe. In the United States (the major oat producer of the world), its production volume exceeds all other grains except corn and wheat. Oat is classified according to planting seasons as winter or spring oats. More than 95 percent of the oat grown commercially is used as pasturage and hay crop. It is an especially nutritious feed for horses. Oat flour does not contain gluten, the proteinlike substance which makes the bread dough cohesive and it is, therefore, not suitable for breadmaking. However, it is used by the food industry as an additive in certain dairy products (e.g., in ice cream). For direct human consumption, oat is usually processed in the form of rolled oats, flakes, or meal, and it is used chiefly as breakfast food. (The popular English porridge is oatmeal cooked in milk.) Oat is primarily a carbohydrate food, but it contains considerable amounts of plant proteins and other nutrients. There are many different brand cereals which use oats. The manner in which they are processed is the key, along with the ingredients, to their nutritional value, and the buyer can decipher this by reading the label.

ORGANIC (fr. L. *organum*, akin to Gk. *ergon* work, and fr. Gk. *organon*, lit. tool, instrument; lit. something that is alive, functioning)

In association with health foods and related subjects, the word *organic* is used as "relating to, or derived from, living organisms," and expresses and defines the idea and concept of *natural* vs. *artificial*. For instance, "organic vegetables" is an illogical misnomer since there are no inorganic vegetables. In this context, however, *organic* denotes the method of producing and processing the vegetables. See: **Organic Farming and Gardening.**

ORGANIC FARMING AND GARDENING

The growing and cultivating of plants in, and the raising and breeding of livestock on, soil free of chemical fertilizers, pesticides, and herbicides. The soil's fertility, texture, and temperature should be maintained and restored by its own natural and readily decomposable and absorbable material, that is, natural compost (e.g., animal manure and other decayed organic matter). After the use of chemical fertilizers spread around the world, some agronomists feared that this would adversely affect the soil, degenerate the plants, and deprive them of their nutritional values. One of the earliest advocates of abandoning artificial (chemical) fertilizers and returning to the old methods was Sir Albert Howard, a British government agronomist stationed in India. He attempted to prove that plants grown in soil fertilized with chemicals are inferior in nutrients. His claims, however, have not been substantiated by scientific evidence.

Organic farming and gardening was started in this country in the early forties by the late Jerome I. Rodale, who named this type of soil cultivating and crop raising "organic." He claimed that all plants lose nutritional values when grown in soil treated with chemical fertilizers. (This has not been proven scientifically.) Soil is similar to a living organism, therefore, only animal or vegetable fertilizers will preserve its vitality. (He also advocated eating raw food.) Today, there are many organic farms and gardens supplying the health food stores and the general market with their produce, either in fresh condition or canned and packaged without chemical additives. See: **Organic Foods, Biodynamic Farming.**

ORGANIC FOODS

Any foodstuff, such as vegetables and fruits, grown in soil fertilized with natural compost only (i.e., animal manure and other decayed organic matter), and without the use of any chemical herbicides and pesticides; and the meat and other products of animals that were not exposed to drugs, chemicals, and commercially processed fodder usually given to livestock, and preferably raised and bred on organic farms.

Claims that organically grown fruits and vegetables have more nutrients and have, therefore, greater nutritional values, have not been substantiated by evidence. It is, however, generally true that organic fruits and vegetables, if grown proficiently and harvested in ripe condition, will taste better than the conventional kind. Since organically grown fruits and vegetables are not cultivated under "controlled" but under natural conditions, the end product may not always be flawless, and the same species may vary in size and shape.

The meat of organically raised animals (cattle, sheep, pigs, and poultry) tastes no better than that of ordinary livestock but it generally tends to be leaner. Claims for better and higher nutritional values have not been proven.

It is possible, though there is no proof for the claim, that organically grown plants and the meat of organically raised animals are free of absorbed chemicals. See: **Organic Farming and Gardening, Natural Foods.**

ORGANIC PEANUT BUTTER (also called "Natural Peanut Butter")

It is made from skinned, ground, and roasted peanuts grown on organic farms, and without any artificial additives. Because organic peanut butter is not homogenized, its oil content will separate from the bulk material and, therefore, it requires mixing before use. It has no better nutritional value than the ordinary peanut butter. Some brands contain added defatted wheat germs, chiefly to enhance the flavor. The wheat germs are defatted in order not to increase the relatively high calorie content of the peanut butter. Organic peanut butter is available in health food stores. See: **Peanut.**

ORGAN MEATS (also called "Glandular meats")

The generic name used by health food advocates for the internal organs of animals, such as the brain, thymus (known as sweetbread) heart, lung, liver, kidney, and the bone marrow. Food of animal origin (e.g., meat, fish, fowl, dairy products) is the best source of high-quality proteins containing all the essential amino acids. However, the internal organs are in addition very rich in minerals, many vitamins, and other vital nutrients. (Vitamin D, for instance, except for insignificant amounts in mushrooms, can only be obtained from animal sources, chiefly from the liver.) Organ meats are very popular in many countries and are not only considered nutritious delicacies but, prepared in many different ways, are part of the regular daily diet. In the United States they are generally regarded as low-grade meat products and are, with the exception of the liver, rarely consumed. To counteract this rather emotionally motivated avoidance nutritionists recommend "disguising" organ meats by mixing them into ground meats, stews, and soups.

OXIDATION

A chemical reaction in which oxygen (air) is combined with an element or compound and thus causing certain changes. For instance, oxidation in foods, especially in fatty foods, will result in losses of the nutritive values and flavor, unpleasant odor, and discoloration. Rancidity is the form of oxidation which affects chiefly fats and oils, particularly those of animal origin. Hydrogenation of fats and oils will prevent rancidity for a longer period of time. Vegetable oils contain substances which have a resistance to oxidation and delay the onset of rancidity. Keeping fatty foods, fats and oils in a cool and dark place in tightly closed containers, thus preventing contact with air, will forestall oxidation. In carbohydrate foods, such as vegetables and fruits, oxidation causes discoloration and destruction of the texture. Various chemicals, called antioxidants, are added to many commercially processed foods in order to prevent oxidation. See: **Preservatives.**

PASTEURIZATION

A process, developed by the French chemist and bacteriologist Louis Pasteur (1822–1895), whereby a liquid is heated for 30 minutes to a temperature of 145° F, then cooled quickly to below 50° F. This partial sterilization process, widely used in the milk industry as a sanitary measure, will destroy and delay the development of disease-causing bacteria, but it also will adversely affect practically all nutritive substances inherent in milk. Pasteurized milk is free of pathogenic organisms, but it contains less proteins, vitamins, minerals, and enzymes than the unprocessed, fresh milk. See: Subentry on Certified Raw Milk under **Milk.**

PEANUT

The edible oily seed of an annual leguminous plant (*Arachis hypogaea*), native to South America, but now widely cultivated in many tropical, subtropical, and temperate regions, especially in India and China. The plant's unusual habit is to push its elongated stalk (vine) which carries the seed vessel, into the ground where the vessel ripens into a pod usually containing two seeds. The peanut (also called earthnut, groundnut) is a highly nutritious food, rich in proteins, minerals, vitamins of the B complex, and also contains vitamin E. Its by-products, especially oil and flour, are also important commercially and are used by the food and chemical industries. Health food stores carry raw and roasted peanuts grown on organic farms, as well as peanut oil, flour, and butter which are unadulterated and contain no artificial additives. See: **Organic Peanut Butter** and subentry on Vegetable Oils under **Fats and Oils.**

PHOTOSYNTHESIS (fr. Gk. *photōs* light, and *synthesis* fr. Gk. *syn* together and *tithenai* to put)

A process whereby plants, utilizing the radiant energy of the sunlight, manufacture carbohydrates in their chlorophyll-containing tissues. Photosynthesis is considered as the ultimate source of energy for all living beings. In plants, water is carried to leaves which absorb carbon dioxide from the air. With the aid of sunlight, the green pigment (chlorophyll) in the plant converts the water and carbon dioxide into carbohydrates (sugars) through a series of complex processes. Some of these sugars are utilized by the plant for immediate energy; some are stored in various parts of the plant; others are converted into starches and deposited, chiefly in the seeds, roots and tubers, for future use. During photosynthesis, plants release oxygen which provides most of the atmospheric oxygen vital to human and animal respiration which, in turn, releases the carbon dioxide necessary for photosynthesis in plants. See: **Carbohydrates.**

POULTRY

Domesticated birds, mainly chicken, turkey, goose, and duck, raised for food (meat and egg). Chicken is the chief poultry bird. It originated probably in Southwest Asia and has been domesticated for over 3,000 years. Chickens are classified either according to their breeding places (e.g., American, Mediterranean, Asian), or according to the various breeds (e.g., Brahmas, Cornish, Jersey Black Giants raised primarily for meat; Leghorns, Anconas raised mainly for eggs; and the American dual-purpose breeds, the Plymouth Rock, Rhode Island Red, New Hampshire, and Wyandotte). Chicken was introduced to the New World by the Spanish, but the turkey is indigenous to the Americas, and the domestic variety is a descendant of the Mexican wild turkey. Wild turkey was served at the first Thanksgiving dinner, and later became the symbol and main food of festivities in the United States.

The goose, a migratory swimming bird related to the duck and the swan, exists in many parts of the world; 4,000 years ago it was a sacred bird to the Egyptians; and early Romans were known to have domesticated geese. Goose meat is popular in countries of south and east Europe, the Mediterranean, and Asia. In certain countries, especially in France and Hungary, geese are forcibly fed to fatten and enlarge the liver which, baked or made into a paste (pâté de foie gras), is considered a great delicacy.

The different species of duck, also a migratory swimming bird, are indigenous to North and South America, Europe, and Asia. The mallard (found in all these parts of the world) is the ancestor of all domestic breeds. Ducks and geese are raised for meat, and their feathers used for pillow stuffing. In many countries both the wild duck and the wild goose are regarded as game fowl and are hunted.

The true game birds are the various species of the pheasant (related to the turkey), partridge, guinea fowl, and grouse, though certain varieties of the pheasant and guinea fowl are domesticated in many parts of the world.

All poultry meat is a good source of the complete proteins (chicken and turkey having slightly more than beef and veal), is rich in minerals (e.g., phosphorus, calcium, iron), and contains several vitamins of the B complex (e.g., B_1, B_2, niacin). Poultry has more unsaturated fatty acids and less saturated ones than meat. The commercial breeding and processing of poultry is under strict governmental regulation and, contrary to widespread belief, the use of hormones to induce quick weight gain is outlawed.

PRESERVATIVES

Chemical substances added to various food products that protect against spoilage, discoloration, and decay by destroying or inhibiting the growth of microorganisms. Food preservation has been practiced throughout the centuries by sun-drying and smoking fish and meat; salting and smoking meat; sun-drying fruits and vegetables; and soaking certain foods in plant juices. At the beginning of the last century canning, the "mechanical" food preservation, was invented and became a large industry. The principles of commercial and domestic canning of foods are the same: precooking, or pretreating (spicing, salting), air-tight sealing of the container, and heating. This procedure usually causes variable losses in the nutrients and changes in the taste. With the advancement of technology, a great variety of chemical substances were dis-

covered or synthetized that had preservative properties, and were added to fresh foods, and to most
canned foods as well. Many chemicals are used to
inhibit the growth of bacteria and molds that
thrive in a moist and warm environment. Protein
and carbohydrate foods that have a high moisture
content are especially susceptible to contamination
by microorganisms (e.g., meat and dairy products,
flour and baked products, vegetables and fruits),
while seeds, cereal grains, and nuts do not need
this type of preservative since their moisture content is low. All animal fats and oils become rapidly
rancid and will consequently develop an unpleasant odor and taste. This process is called oxidation.
It is not caused by microorganisms but by oxygen
in the air, the temperature, or by inherent enzymes
producing chemical changes. Such oxidation can
also affect certain carbohydrate foods causing discoloration, but it has little or no effect on the taste
and odor (e.g., sliced fruits and vegetables will
turn brown when exposed to air). To prevent oxidation and preserve freshness, various chemicals,
called antioxidants, are added to such foodstuffs.
Many foods and drinks contain metals (naturally
occurring minerals), or come in contact with
metals during processing (e.g., canned foods).
These minerals, not by themselves but acting as
chemical catalysts, will cause discoloration, loss of
flavor, and deterioration of the foods, or cloudiness
in soft drinks. To prevent this, several chemical
substances, called chelating (fr. Gk. *chēlē*, claw)

or sequestering (fr. L. *sequestare* to set apart) agents, are added to such foodstuffs to render the minerals chemically inactive. Other chemical substances, called polyhydric alcohols, are added to foods in order to preserve their moist texture and freshness. These chemicals absorb and retain water, and can also control the viscosity of the food material (e.g., keeping cakes or certain kinds of confection moist or soft and chewy.) The effectiveness of almost all preservatives used by the food industry is limited to a relatively short period of time. Today, practically every commercially processed fresh and canned food contains chemical preservatives. See: Additives.

PROTEIN (fr. Gk. *proteios* primary, fr. Gk. *protos* first; lit. at the first place)

Any one of a great variety of very complex organic compounds occurring in plants and animals. Proteins are combinations of amino acids containing the elements carbon, hydrogen, oxygen, and nitrogen, and in varying degrees some other elements such as sulphur, iron, phosphorus, and iodine. Proteins are the essential constituents of all living cells. Of all organic substances in the protoplasm (the fundamental material of which all living things are composed) protein occurs in the greatest quantity. Protein is the source, in many cases the only source, of nitrogen which is vital to the development, growth, and replacement of all tissues. Proteins also serve as important sources of energy. Since every cell contains proteins (even the bones and teeth were originally proteins), protein is regarded as the basic substance of life.

No protein has been synthetized and, though many proteins have been isolated in crystalline form, because of their extreme complexity and diversity, such proteins are chemically not pure. Of the more than 30 known amino acids composing the structure of proteins, 22 have been identified. The human body is able to manufacture in the digestive tract 14 of these 22 amino acids, but only if the other 8 (which have been designated as indispensable) are supplied in the food. These 8 essential amino acids are isoleucine, leucine, lysine, methionine, phenylalanine, tryptophane, threonine, and valine. In a broader sense, two additional amino acids, arginine and histidine, are also "essential" since the body is not able to produce them fast enough to ensure a ready and adequate supply.

Proteins are considered as the most vital of all nutrients. The nutritive value of a protein, however, depends on the combination of the amino acids. Proteins containing the highest percentages of the essential amino acids are called "complete" or "first class" proteins. Proteins of animal origin are superior in quality and are biologically more active than those of plant origin. Rich sources of complete proteins are meat, organ meats (e.g., liver), dairy products (e.g., milk, cheese, eggs), seafood (e.g., fish, oysters). Vegetable proteins are incomplete. The proteins in soybean become complete if the soybean is heated, but they are still not equivalent in quality to the proteins of animal origin. Brewer's yeast, sunflower seeds, peanuts, peanut flour, and wheat germ are good sources of vegetable proteins. Nutritionists recommend that at least two thirds of the daily protein intake should be animal protein, and they consider a high-protein and low-carbohydrate diet as essential to good health. The Food and Nutrition Board of the National Research Council recommends 60–65 grams of daily protein intake for men, and 50 grams for women. These "officially" suggested daily amounts of proteins, however, are regarded by many nutritionists as insufficient and they recommend twice the amount. (Four ounces of liver contains about 25 grams of complete proteins; one half of a cup of cottage cheese about 20 grams, and four ounces of hamburger about 20 grams.)

PROTEIN CONCENTRATE, WHOLE FISH

The idea of utilizing high-quality fish protein to alleviate the serious problem of protein deficiency in the world was conceived several decades ago.

It was proposed to convert the vast amounts of readily available but otherwise not edible fish into a low cost complete protein dietary supplement.

Whole fish protein concentrate is manufactured by drying and grinding the whole fish (i.e., head, skin, bones, and viscera) into a fine powder after the oils and fats have been extracted. In the United States it is only recently that the Food and Drug Administration has approved the use of such protein concentrate for human consumption but only as a food additive. Whole fish protein concentrate in the United States cannot be made from so-called "trash fish" (nonfood fish) but only from selected species proven to be nontoxic; the concentrate must be deodorized (nondeodorized fish protein concentrate is used as feed for livestock, especially for poultry). Whole fish protein concentrate cannot be used in commercially processed foods but only in home cooking and baking. This ruling is primarily for the benefit of those people who would object to eating derivatives of whole fish, though there are concentrates made from eviscerated fish. Whole fish protein concentrate is one of the most condensed and least expensive source of high-quality proteins. (A half ounce provides the protein value of two and a half ounces of steak.) It can be used in baking (mixed into the flour), in sauces, and in certain soups. It can be stored without refrigeration for several months. See: **Protein Preparations.**

PROTEIN HYDROLYSATES

A mixture of various amino acids produced by splitting proteins, both of plant and animal origin, with enzyme, acid, or alkali. In the form of their constituent amino acids, these "predigested" proteins have the same nutritional values as the original material. Such preparations are used in special diets if there is a sensitivity (e.g., allergic reaction) to ordinary food proteins, or are added to certain foods (e.g., dried soup mixtures) to provide readily digestible proteins.

PROTEIN PREPARATIONS

Dietary food supplement products containing complete proteins, that is, all the essential amino acids which are indispensable but cannot be manufactured in the body and must, therefore, be supplied in food. Most preparations contain many additional amino acids. The protein is usually derived from yeast, nonfat milk, eggs, meat, liver, fish, soybean, and wheat germ, and in some products they are obtained entirely from sea animals and vegetables. Many products also contain the vitamins of the B complex and several minerals in various amounts. For vegetarians who may have difficulty in obtaining the necessary proteins in the usual diet, such preparations are made from vegetable sources only (e.g., soybean, wheat germ, cotton seed). Protein preparations supply high energy and are used as a food supplement for augmenting muscle strength. All these products are available at health food stores either in powder form (to be added to ordinary food or mixed into drinks), or as tablets, or as ready-to-eat foods such as wafers, cookies, candy bars, and so forth. See: **Protein Concentrate, Whole Fish.**

RAW FOOD

It is not exactly known when man first applied fire to food. It is however assumed that heating of food became customary among all peoples comparatively late in the long history of mankind. Today, most foodstuffs (and practically all protein foods consumed) come into contact with heat in one way or another. Heating, especially extensive cooking, will affect most nutrients in food. This may manifest itself in the complete or partial destruction of a certain nutrient and in changes in the metabolic processes. For instance, it is known that strong heat will destroy most proteins, but the total effect of any heat on proteins has still not been precisely determined. However, it is proven that the heating of protein will definitely lower its digestibility and make it biologically less effective (e.g., raw meat is digested in about one to two hours, while well-done, fried, or roasted meat will require four hours of digestion). In spite of heating (cooking) many foodstuffs, most of the necessary vitamins, minerals, and enzymes can be obtained by eating fresh fruits, vegetables, and dairy products (including pasteurized milk). Since nearly all of the proteins are supplied in foods of animal origin that are almost always exposed to heating, nutritionists recommend the regular consumption of unprocessed and uncooked protein foods, such as raw milk and eggs, and other dairy products, oysters and clams and, from inspected sources, raw fish (dried, marinated) and beef (steak tartar).

RICE

An annual, Asiatic cereal plant (*Oryza sativa*) of the Grass family, originating probably in the moist, subtropical regions of river deltas. It has been cultivated in China for more than 4,000 years from where it was introduced to India, Japan, and other countries. Thousands of strains are known, and several varieties have been developed that are acclimatized to, and are now cultivated in, temperate climates in many parts of the world, including the

United States. Rice is the most important commodity in the Orient, and its seeds constitute the basic food for almost half of the world's population. It is also utilized in many other ways, for example, the straw serves as a weaving and packaging material and, mixed with bran and meal, as animal feed; from the grain alcoholic beverages (saki, raki) are distilled.

Rice also provides many basic materials to food, chemical, and other industries. Rice is a carbohydrate food, the grain consisting mainly of starch. Its nutritional value is in the various inner layers of its bran. Threshing by hand (as it has been practiced for centuries), or milling (polishing) the rice (as it is done now by machines), separates the grain from the bran, thus removing most of the nutrients. (The polished or white rice is the basic material of laundry starches and dusting powder.) The unpolished or natural rice is the unprocessed whole grain containing all the inherent nutritive substances and, because of its color, is usually called "brown rice." The removed and separated inner layers of the rice bran are called "rice polishing," a product rich in thiamine (vitamin B_1). See: **Tikitiki.**

ROSE HIP

The ripe, "false" fruit of the rose that remains after the petals have fallen off. It consists of a fleshy pod which contains numerous seeds. The hip of the dog rose (*Rosa canina*) is used in pharmacy. Rose hips are rich in vitamin C. Certain varieties (e.g., *Rosa laxa*, a white rose) may yield at peak maturity up to 5,000 milligrams of vitamin C per 100 grams of rose hip. With the onset of cold weather, the vitamin C content decreases rapidly. Rose hip extract is used as a food supplement, and is available in liquid, tablet, and powdered form. Fresh rose hips prepared as preserves or jams, or dried and used as a drink (tea), have always been popular in central and northern European countries and can usually be obtained in this country in stores specializing in imported food or in health food shops.

ROYAL JELLY

A viscid, honeylike secretion of the pharyngeal glands located close to the mouth in the honeybee. Royal jelly contains pantothenic acid and some other vitamins of the B complex, as well as other nutrients essential to the development and sustenance of the bee. It is fed to all young larvae and to all queen larvae in the bee colonies. The widely publicized claims of rejuvenating and other extraordinary beneficial effects of the royal jelly in humans have not been proven. Pure royal jelly is available in capsules, mixed with vitamins, or added to honey and other foods. It is also used in various cosmetic preparations.

RYE

A hardy, annual cereal (grain) plant (*Secale cereale*) of the Grass family. Rye was probably domesticated later than wheat and the other staple grains. In colder climates and where the soil is too poor to produce a good crop of wheat, rye is the preferred grain because it grows well in such soil and can withstand the cold. It became one of the main staple grains of northern Europe. Rye is still an important crop in Europe, not only for human consumption but also as a feed for livestock, especially in the USSR, which leads the world in the production of rye. Rye is particularly susceptible to a disease caused by a poisonous fungus (ergot) which affects and finally replaces the seed of the rye (and other cereal grasses). Drugs derived from this fungus are used in medicine (e.g., to arrest internal bleedings, to hasten labor). However, eating bread made from fungus infected rye flour may cause severe poisoning.

The original "black bread" (Schwarzbrot, or pumpernickel) of the North European Germanic peoples was made from the whole grain flour of rye. The rye bread sold today, however, usually contains more processed white wheat flour than rye flour. The commercial pumpernickel breads are dark mainly because they are colored with burnt sugar (caramel coloring). Alcoholic beverages, such as gin and whisky are distilled from rye grains. Rye, as are all grains, is primarily a carbohydrate food, but its whole grain contains many valuable nutrients and it is believed to be less fattening than wheat. In the United States, rye is used chiefly as feed for animals, and as a cover crop, but in north and central European countries rye flour is much used in breadmaking.

SAGO (fr. Malay *sagu* sago palm)

An edible powdered or granulated starchy food prepared from the stem of various East Indian and Malaysian palms especially the *Metroxylon sago*). Sago is an important part of the diet in India. Some of it is exported and used by the food industry (mainly in puddings and in similar premixed foods), and by the textile industry (as a fabric stiffener). A similar starch product obtained from the tubers and stems of a subtropical American palmlike plant (*Zamia floridana*) is the easily digestible *arrowroot*, usually called sago. It is widely used by the food industry as a thickener in soups, puddings, and other foods. Sago is a carbohydrate food. See: **Tapioca.**

SAFFLOWER

An herb (*Carthamus tinctorius*) having a large red or orange colored head bearing oil-rich seeds. It belongs to the same family (the *Compositae*) as the sunflower. It is widely grown in South Asia and in the Mediterranean region. The extracted oil is used in cooking and baking. Formerly, a reddish liquid prepared from the head of the flower was used as a dyestuff. See: Subentry on *Vegetable Oils* under Fats and Oils.

ST. JOHN'S BREAD

The fruit (legume) of a Mediterranean evergreen tree (*Ceratonia siliqua*) which, according to a Christian legend, was the food of St. John the Baptist during his wanderings in the wilderness. Because of its sweet and pleasant taste, the dried legume is eaten as a delicacy, mainly by children, in the Mediterranean and other European countries. Although some health food stores carry St. John's Bread, it is mainly available in ethnic, especially Eastern and Southern European grocery stores. See: Carob Powder.

SALT

Regular Salt

A crystalline compound of sodium and chlorine, abundant in nature. It constitutes a very important part of the diet, both of men and animals. Common salt (sodium chloride) is widely used for seasoning or preserving food. Most commercially available brands of salt are iodized and because of this are preferable to plain table salt. (See the subentry on Iodine under **Minerals**.)

It is believed that salt is a contributing factor to several diseases and disorders (e.g., it increases blood pressure; it causes fluid retention in the body). In such cases, it is generally recommended that the salt intake should be reduced. Many people advocate the complete elimination of salt from the daily diet as being unnecessary and harmful. Although salt is found in many foodstuffs (e.g., meats, raw vegetables, and fruits), excluding salt indiscriminately from the daily diet may cause adverse reactions since salt is essential to many metabolic and physiological processes.

Sea Salt

Common salt (sodium chloride) obtained by evaporation of sea water, also called "bay salt";

it contains iodine and is said to be generally more valuable as a seasoning than mined salt (rock salt) because of its iodine content.

SEAFOOD

The collective name of all foods obtained from marine animals: fish and shellfish. The seas, lakes, and rivers have provided man with food since prehistoric times, and fisheries were of great commercial importance in the earliest civilizations. Today, around 100 billion pounds of fish are caught yearly by the fishing nations of the world, led by Japan. Seafood comprises about one tenth of the world's flesh foods. Fish by-products include crude oil, fish liver oils, fish meal (used for feeding poultry and other livestock and as fertilizer), glue, and gelatine.

Among the chief food fishes are the tuna, salmon, herring, cod, haddock, halibut, mackerel, flounder, sole, bluefish, trout, carp; mollusks such as oyster, clam, scallop, and squid; and crustaceans which include shrimp, crab, and lobster. Seafood is an excellent source of the biologically highly effective complete proteins (one ounce of fish is, or two shrimps of medium size are, equal in protein value to one ounce of meat), and it is rich in several vitamins (e.g., vitamins A, B_1, B_6, niacin, choline). Some fish (e.g., salmon) and especially the fish liver oils are the best food sources of the vitamins D and A. Raw clams and oysters also contain vitamin C. Minerals (e.g., iodine, iron, phosphorus) are present in all seafoods; lobster is the richest source of the trace mineral cobalt. Herring, salmon, eel, mackerel, and sturgeon have more fat than other fish and shellfish, but actually all seafood is low in fat content. Fish liver oil and fat are high in unsaturated fatty acids.

Fish and shellfish are marketed fresh, canned, dried and smoked, pickled, and frozen. Fresh seafood spoils quickly and must be refrigerated and consumed promptly after being taken from the water. It can be prepared in many ways, for example, boiled, broiled, fried, baked, cooked, or steamed, but oysters and fish eggs (caviar) are eaten raw and both are considered by many people as great delicacies. In several countries (e.g., Japan, Peru) certain fishes are also consumed raw, sometimes marinated and usually served with a sauce. See: subentry on Fish Liver Oils under Fats and Oils.

SEAWEED

General

The common name of multicellular marine algae (pl. of L. *alga* seaweed), the most primitive group of plants, lacking true roots, stems, leaves, and flowers. They are the chief aquatic plant life in the seas and fresh waters, and constitute the main food supply for all marine animals and, indirectly, for many land animals. Algae have chlorophyll and the capacity of supplying oxygen through photosynthesis. The gelatinous substance (agar) obtained from seaweeds is used in the food and other industries. Seaweeds are rich in iodine, and also contain other minerals, vitamins, and proteins. An important part of the diet of most countries of the Far East and the Pacific, seaweeds are widely used as vegetables and in soups, and are eaten cooked, roasted, or dehydrated. Species of the red algae are "farmed" for food in Japan and China. Large scale farming of seaweed has been considered in several countries to supplement the production of land agriculture, and as a source of food and oxygen in space travel.

Dulse

Any of the several harsh-textured red seaweeds (especially *Rhodymenia palmata*) usually found in northern latitudes and used mostly as food seasoning. They are a rich source of iodine.

Kelp

The generic name of various large brown seaweeds, especially abundant in Japan, but also found on the west coast of the United States (especially *Macrocystis pyrifera*). Like other seaweeds, kelps are rich in iodine and other minerals, and contain vitamins and proteins. The extracted minerals from the ashes of burned kelp are used in various industries (e.g., chemical reagents), and in agriculture (e.g., fodder, fertilizer). Kelp also serves as a source for vitamin and mineral preparations. In Japan, various foods known as *kombu* are made from kelp. In this country, dehydrated kelp, dulse, and sea lettuce (*Ulva*) are occasionally eaten, but are not popular. Health food stores carry kelp in tablet form and, because of its high iodine content, as a seasoning powder to replace the common rock salt.

SEEDS

The grains or ripened ovules of plants of the highest order. The seeds consist of the germ or embryo (the reproductive part of the seeds), the endosperm (containing the stored food material for the plant), and the outer cover. In some cases the outer cover is a hard shell (e.g., coconut, Brazil nut), in other cases it is brittle (e.g., the bran of various cereal grains). Seeds are often confused with nuts and the fruits enclosing them. The size of seeds may vary from the minute dustlike seeds of most flowers to the largest seed contained in the coconut. Seeds, which are usually referred to as "nuts," were among the first food plants eaten by man. Various seeds and food products made from them are considered as staple food for man and animals in many countries.

Seeds can be eaten raw or dried, and are sometimes roasted (e.g., the "nuts," wheat germ, sunflower seed); some types of seeds, especially those of the leguminous plants (e.g., beans, peas) are consumed usually cooked; and some seeds are used as seasonings (e.g., caraway, dill). All seeds have high nutritive values. They are rich in oil containing unsaturated fatty acids, vitamin E, several vitamins of the B complex, many minerals, and also proteins. Most seeds are viable for many years, and will not germinate if kept in closed containers in a cool and dry place. After germination of the seed, the vitamin content of the very young plant increases (except for vitamin E), but the oil content decreases. Germinated seeds (i.e., sprouts) are a popular vegetable supplement in many countries. Nutritionists recommend the consumption of seeds (and nuts) as a snack instead of sweet and starchy foods. Seeds and seed products (e.g., flour, paste, confections) are available at health food stores. See: **Nuts, Sunflower Seeds, Sesame Seeds, Wheat Germ, Sprouts.**

SEMOLINA (fr. It. *semola* bran)

A flour made from the purified middlings (the bran and other nutritive constituents) of the durum wheat. However, the flour is usually refined and bleached which adversely affects its nutritional value. Semolina flour is used chiefly in the manufacture of spaghetti, macaroni, and vermicelli. See: **Wheat, Bran.**

SESAME SEEDS (fr. L. *sesamum*, fr. Gk. *sesamon*, akin to Ar. *simsim*)

The edible and very oil-rich (about 50 percent) seeds of East Indian herbs (*Sesamum indicum* and *S. orientale*). The extracted oil is used in cooking, or as a salad oil, in many countries from the Far East to Africa and the Mediterranean regions. The seeds are ground into a paste which is used as a base for candies and pastries and also as a shortening. Because of their soothing properties for irritation and inflammation, the seeds are useful in dysentery. In some countries, sesame oil is used as an additive to margarine. Sesame seeds are rich in proteins, minerals, and unsaturated fatty acids. They are also a good source of the vitamin B complex. See: Subentry on Vegetable Oils under **Fats and Oils.**

SHORTENING

An edible fat, made from vegetable oils, sometimes with the addition of animal fat, and used in cooking, frying, and baking. In the manufacturing process, hydrogenation is used to change the usually liquid consistency of the basic fats and oils into a hardened product. Hydrogenation not only condenses the fats and oils but renders them less susceptible to rancidity and thereby expands their shelf life. Shortenings remain fresh for a long period of time even without refrigeration. This process, however, destroys many nutrients in the fats and oils, thus reducing the nutritive values of the shortenings. Nearly all shortenings contain chemical preservatives (antioxidants), and some other additives. Shortenings made from vegetable oils contain considerably more saturated and less unsaturated fatty acids than do fresh vegetable oils, and they have approximately the same amounts of the saturated and unsaturated fatty acids as margarine. Shortening is relatively high in calories as are all fats and oils.

SORGHUM

Any of the economically important tall, coarse annual drought-resistant plants of the Grass family, especially the widely cultivated common sorghum (*Sorghum vulgare*). Originating probably in Africa, numerous types of sorghum are now also grown in Asia (especially in India and China), in the Mediterranean regions, in southern Europe, and in America. Sorghum yields a great variety of products used in agriculture and industry. In the United States, sorghum is utilized mainly as forage and feed grain for livestock. The sweet varieties (sorgos) yield a syrup which resembles cane syrup but which contains a good deal of simple sugar. Sorghum meal as an additive in cooking and baking, and sorghum syrup for sweetening are available in health food stores.

SOFT DRINKS

The common name for drinks not containing alcohol. There is a great variety of such drinks. Several brands contain extracts from coca leaves and kola nuts, sugar, and aromatic substances. Other brands contain natural or artificial fruit or other flavors, coloring agents, and preservatives. To some soft drinks, synthetic vitamins (usually vitamin C) are added. Many brands are manufactured with carbonated water. Soft drinks have no nutritional values, and most physicians, nutritionists, and dentists consider the regular drinking of soft drinks containing coca and kola extracts and sugar, especially by children, as undesirable because of the various adverse effects it may cause to the teeth, and the nervous and digestive systems. See: **Cola Drinks.**

SOYBEAN (fr. D. *Soya,* fr. J. *shōyu,* fr. Ch. *chiang yu,* lit. soybean oil)

A hairy, leguminous Asiatic plant (*Glycine max,* or *G. soja*), native to the tropical and warmer regions of the Far East where, next to rice, it is a principal crop. It has been widely cultivated there for more than 5,000 years, chiefly for its oil-rich, protein containing seeds, and as a forage. In the diet of the East, which consists mainly of rice, soybean is a major factor in preventing nutritional deficiencies by providing nutrients lacking in rice. Many of the more than 2,500 varieties are now also grown and cultivated in Europe and North America. In the Orient, soybeans are used in many forms, for example, as cooking oil, sauces, raw or cooked sprouts, fresh or dried as vegetable, curdled as soy cheese and soy "milk." Soybean oil, flour, and other derivatives are also used in food, chemical, and other industries. All soybean products are very high in proteins and, if quickly heated for a short time, the quality of the proteins will increase. Soybean is sometimes referred to as the "meat that grows on trees," or as the "poor man's steak." Its protein is not quite equivalent to that of animal origin, but it is still superior to other vegetable proteins. Soybean is low in carbohydrates but rich in minerals and in vitamins (espe-

cially the fresh beans and sprouts). The oil is a
good source of unsaturated fatty acids. There are
a great variety of soybean products on the market
and available in health food stores, for example,
soybean oil for cooking, baking, salad dressings;
sauce for seasoning; green soybeans (canned or
frozen) for vegetable dishes or salads; sprouts
(canned or in jars), flour, a natural and nutritious
additive to other foods; roasted beans. See: Subentry on Vegetable Oils under **Fats and Oils,
Sprouts.**

SPICES

Plant products with a specific taste and/or odor,
used chiefly as seasonings in foods and drinks.
Many spices are also used by the pharmaceutical
industry as flavoring agents in medicines, and by
the cosmetic industry as fragrance in perfumes and
soaps. Spices are the oldest food additives and
have played a significant role in trade and commerce since antiquity. Most originated in tropical
Asia, South America, and the West Indies, but
many spice producing plants now grow in temperate zones. As valuable condiments, spices were
carried from the East by caravans across China
and India to the Near East and the market places
in Europe where they were sold for high prices, or
used as medium of exchange. The spice trade de-
clined in the Middle Ages but was revived and

intensified during the fifteenth, sixteenth, and seventeenth centuries. Because of the lack of refrigeration and difficulties in transportation, certain foods, especially meat products, were heavily salted, or became spoiled. Thus spices were needed not only to render the bland European diet more tasty, but also to be used as preservatives. The high price of spices and the fact that most overland routes from Asia were cut off were partly responsible for the bitter rivalry of the European powers in their competitive search for new trade routes across the Oceans. Spices were valuable articles of commerce, and wars among the European powers were fought for the control of the major spice producing areas.

Spices are used in various forms: the seeds of a plant (e.g., caraway); the dried berries (e.g., black pepper); the roots (e.g., horseradish); the bulb (e.g., garlic); the bark (e.g., cinnamon); the pod (e.g., green pepper). However, most spices are available, and more commonly used, in convenient powder form, or as essential oils extracted from the plants. Several spices have been chemically synthetized and are used by the food industry as flavoring agents. See: **Flavoring Agents, Herbs.**

SPROUTS

The immature outgrowth from a plant, or the shoot from its germinated seed, especially the edible sprouts of leguminous and grain producing plants (e.g., all types of beans and the related peas, alfalfa, lentil, wheat, rye, corn, millet). During the germination period, practically all nutritive substances in the seeds increase, and several of them are converted into more easily digestible forms (e.g., much of the starch in the soybean is reduced to simple sugars in the sprout). This increase of nutrients is especial to the species, and may fluctuate according to the conditions and the length of the germination period. After reaching optimum growth, the sprouts must be refrigerated in order to prevent their deterioration. Most sprouts can be eaten either raw or cooked, and added to almost any other food. Sprouts are part of the daily diet in many countries of the Orient. In this country, only a few varieties are grown for consumption and are available, fresh, canned or dehydrated (dried) in health food stores and in oriental groceries. See: **Alfalfa, Soybean, Wheat Germ.**

STABILIZERS AND THICKENERS
Substances extracted from plants, or obtained by chemical synthesis, that are added to various foods and drinks in order to bind together (stabilize) the liquid and solid parts of certain foods, and to prevent the evaporation of flavoring oils; or else to

add "body" or bulkiness (thickness) to foods and drinks.

Seaweed and gum extracted from trees were used for many centuries as thickeners and stabilizers in home cooking. The ever growing production of all types of commercially processed food and drink requires today a greater variety and wider usage of stabilizers and thickeners. For instance, the chocolate particles in chocolate milk would separate from the milk without a stabilizer which, by altering the viscosity of the milk, keeps the chocolate particles suspended; and the excess water in ice cream would freeze into small granules without the addition of a stabilizer. Thickeners, when added to soups, puddings, cheese spreads, cake toppings, and sauces, create the desirable consistency in these and many other foods; they also add fullness to sugarless diet drinks. Most stabilizers and thickeners used by the food industry are extracted from natural sources, that is, seaweeds, trees, and seeds; some of them are chemically modified, but only a few are entirely synthetized products. The addition of any such agent to foods and drinks, whether extracted from natural sources or chemically synthetized, must be stated on the product's package or label. See: **Additives.**

STARCH

A colorless, tasteless complex carbohydrate substance, produced by plants through photosynthesis first as sugar which is then converted into starch and stored in the seeds, roots, stems, and flowers as food for the plants. It plays an important role in the biochemistry of plants and animals, and it is one of the major foodstuffs for men and animals. It is abundant in all grains, grain products, tubers (e.g., potatoes), and dried legumes. Starch, prepared chiefly from corn, potatoes, and rice, has many commercial applications and is widely used in the food, chemical, and other industries. In the body, the digestive process converts starch into sugar which supplies energy. Most of the unused sugar is stored in the liver as glycogen ("animal starch") for future needs. Excessive accumulation of starch in the body, however, usually results in obesity. For instance, refined flour made from the endosperm formed within the embryo sac of the whole grain after removal of the bran and germ, which contain the vital nutrients (e.g., vitamins, minerals), is practically "pure" starch without nutrients. Exclusive consumption of such food may cause serious nutritional deficiencies, and other disorders. See: **Carbohydrates, Sugar.**

SUGAR

White Sugar

The most widely used sweetening agent, white sugar is a crystallized, refined carbohydrate substance, obtained primarily from two plants. One is the sugar cane (*Saccharum officinarum*), a tall, perennial tropical plant of the Grass family, native to Asia from where it was introduced to other tropical regions of the world. It is now cultivated in many countries, especially in Cuba, Brazil, and India, which are the major cane sugar producers of the world. The juice is extracted from the cut stalks; then through evaporation of the juice's excess water the brownish colored raw sugar is obtained. (By-products include molasses, rum, feed for livestock.) White sugar is obtained from the raw sugar through a refining process which whitens it and removes the nonsugar components from it.

The other plant is a variety of a beet (*Beta vulgaris*), developed for its sugar content during the nineteenth century, and is now cultivated throughout the temperate zones of the world. It supplies about one third of the world's sugar. The method of extracting the juice from the beet and the subsequent refining processes are similar to those employed in the manufacture of the cane sugar. The beet has no usable by-products. Both the refined white cane and beet sugar are pure sucrose and have no intrinsic nutrients.

Through photosynthesis plants transform carbon, hydrogen, and oxygen into sugars which are then converted into starches and stored in the plants' seeds, roots, stems, and flowers. All sugars fall into three groups: (1) the simple sugars (monosaccharides), that is, glucose and fructose (also called evulose and dextrose) that are quickly absorbed and are present in most fruits, vegetables, honey; (2) the double sugars (disaccharides, the combination of two simple sugars) which are lactose, the milk sugar; maltose which is present in germinating grains and other seeds; and sucrose, the refined white cane and beet sugar; (3) the multiple sugars (polysaccharides, which are the combination of several simple sugars) are found in grain products and dried legumes. Double and multiple sugars require breaking down into simple sugars through digestion before they can be absorbed and utilized as energy, or stored in the livers of people and animals as glycogen ("animal starch") for future use. Other sources of sugar are certain food acids which also provide energy, or are stored in the body. When more sugar is absorbed than can be utilized or stored, the surplus is converted into fat, causing internal and external obesity. Naturally occurring sugars (as in grain products, fruits, honey) usually provide sufficient sugar necessary for energy production. The additional excessive consumption of refined sugar in any form (e.g., in drinks, in baked products, as syrup) may bring on serious disorders. For instance, it disturbs the balance of the nutrients and increases the need for vitamins; accelerates the elevation of the blood-sugar level which is usually followed by a sudden drop causing hypoglycemia (low-blood sugar) inducing an abnormal desire for food ("hunger disease"). White refined sugar is sometimes referred to as "useless calories." See: **Carbohydrates, Starch.**

Raw Sugar (also called "brown sugar," "yellow sugar")

It is basically the same sugar as the highly processed white sugar but, not having been refined, it still retains some small amounts of nutrients. Its nutritional values, however, are negligible and, like refined white sugar, increase the need for vitamins without providing them. For purposes of health, raw sugar is not a replacement for refined white sugar since its actions and effects are the same. Raw sugar, like white sugar, is a double sugar (sucrose), and requires digestion before absorption. Packaged raw sugar for human consumption is available but, unless it has been processed by a reputable manufacturer, it may be contaminated with dirt. Health food stores, however, carry various selected brands of packaged raw sugar.

SUN-DRIED FRUITS

Sun-drying fruits, vegetables, herbs, seeds, and other foods (e.g., fish, meat) has been a common practice since ancient times. Next to salting and smoking, it is one of the oldest forms of food preservation. Sun-drying plant products was especially common in the cold and temperate zones where the availability of fresh produce was restricted or limited by seasonal changes. Fresh fruits contain many vitamins, minerals, and enzymes, and are an excellent source of the readily absorbable simple sugars, fructose and glucose. During the drying process, several of these above nutrients decrease in strength and the sugar content increases (e.g., fresh apricots have a sugar content of approximately 15 percent, but after evaporation of the moisture, the sugar content goes up to over 70 percent). The most popular dried fruits are sliced apples, peaches and apricots, and whole cherries, dates, figs, grapes (raisins), and plums (prunes). Commercially produced dried fruits are usually not sun-dried but dehydrated by the application of chemicals (e.g., treating the fruits with sulphur dioxide gas ["sulphuring"], which is also used in bleaching and as a preservative; sulphuring, however, prevents the loss of vitamin C). Advocates of health foods recommend the consumption only of naturally sun-dried fruits grown on organic farms and free of artificial additives. They also recommend eating dried fruits without cooking them; and if they are soaked in water, drinking the juice. Naturally sun-dried fruits are available in health food stores and are also sold in better groceries and specialty shops.

SUNFLOWER SEEDS

Highly nutritious edible seeds of a North American annual plant (*Helianthus annus*), now cultivated everywhere, especially in Europe and Asia. The seeds, located in the large round center of the flower head, are a staple food for men and animals in many European and Eastern European countries. The tasty dried seeds are eaten or are ground to flour and used, as is the extracted oil, in cooking and baking. The seeds have a high protein content and are rich in vitamins and minerals. Sunflower seeds are available in health food stores in dried form or as a pulver (meal). See: Subentry on Vegetable Oils under **Fats and Oils.**

SURFACE ACTIVE AGENTS

Chemical compounds which, on contact, will alter the surface properties of foodstuffs (or other materials) thereby making possible the mixing of immiscible liquids (e.g., water and oil in salad dressings), or which when absorbed will bind liquids and solids uniformly together (e.g., the oil and solid parts of peanut butter). The surface active compounds include the emulsifiers and foaming agents and serve several purposes (e.g., to increase the volume of baked products and cake mixes; to improve volume and texture of food mixes and fillings; to impart better eating and keeping qualities; and depending on their concentration and combination with other additives, to develop or inhibit foaming, e.g., in soda). Before chemically synthetized compounds were available, lecithin, obtained from natural sources (plants and animals), was used almost exclusively as an emulsifier. Today, all surface active agents used by the food industry are synthetics. Their addition to foods and drinks (e.g., sodas) must be listed on the product's package or label. See: **Additives.**

TAPIOCA (fr. the Brazilian Tupi Indian name *typyóca*) A widely used edible starchy food prepared from the root of the cassava (or manioc) plant (especially the *Manihot esculenta*), which is native to Brazil but is now cultivated in many tropical countries. Cassava has been since ancient times a major source of food for the Indians and it is still an important staple food in the tropics. It is sometimes called bitter cassava because of an acid present in the roots. This, however, is destroyed by cooking. The roots resemble sweet potatoes and are eaten the same way, especially those species yielding roots without acid content. Tapioca is produced as flour, flakes, or fine granules. It is used in puddings, various desserts, and soups. Tapioca is a carbohydrate food. See: Sago.

TEA

The name of a beverage made from the dried leaves of closely related evergreen shrubs (*Thea sinensis, Camellia sinensis,* or *C. thea*). It is indigenous to South China, North East India and, probably, to Japan. Cultivated in China in prehistoric times, tea is believed to have been used first as a medicinal remedy and as a vegetable seasoning. Large scale production of tea began in China and Japan around 900 A.D. The famous tea ceremony (a socio-religious symbol) was introduced to Japan by Chinese Buddhist monks in the fifteenth century. In the early seventeenth century the Dutch brought tea from India to Europe where it became very popular, particularly in Great Britain and Russia. Great Britain obtained an import and trade monopoly from China that was broken in 1834. Thereafter, other tea-growing countries developed into major producers and exporters, for example, India, Japan, Formosa, Indonesia, and Ceylon, which today exports more tea than any other country. Among the largest consumers of tea (outside of Japan, and China, which is the largest tea grower of the world) are the United Kingdom, the USSR, Canada, and Australia. In the United States (also a large importer) the popularity of tea diminished considerably after the Boston Tea Party (1773). More people drink tea and in greater quantity than any other beverage in the world except water.

Tea leaves are hand-picked and dried by rolling and heating; some varieties are fermented (e.g., the black teas); some others are scented with the fragrance of flowers (e.g., lotus, jasmin), but the flavor of the tea is due to inherent volatile oils. Tea contains theine, a slightly bitter crystalline substance (the same occurs in the coffee bean but there it is called caffeine) which has a mild stimulating effect on the nervous and cardio-vascular system. The astringency of tea is due to its tannic acid content. In black teas this is reduced by fermentation.

The caffeine content in coffee and tea depends largely on the variety, the time of harvesting, the processing (drying by air, heat), the roasting method used, and so on. Because a cup of tea contains far less theine (caffeine) than a cup of coffee, it is generally considered as a harmless beverage. Tea has no nutritional values. See: **Coffee, Chocolate, Cola Drinks.**

TIKITIKI (the Japanese name for "Rice Polishing")
An extract or soup made from rice polishing, the inner layers of the rice bran which are removed during the milling process. Because of its high vitamin B_1 content, it is used in Japan in special diets as a neuritis-preventing remedy. See: **Rice.**

VEGETABLE
The common name for a great variety of edible plants, and also for many fruits. Vegetables include the green and leafy parts of plants (e.g., spinach, lettuce, cabbage), the roots and tubers (e.g., carrots, potatoes, beets), the fruits (e.g., tomato, pepper, cucumber, pumpkin), and the seeds (e.g., corn, peas, beans). Mushrooms are generally considered vegetables, although they are actually fungi.

Vegetables are primarily carbohydrate foods consisting mainly of water, sugar, and starches. Their protein content is not significant and the proteins are inferior in quality as compared to animal proteins. The dried legumes (e.g., beans, peas) contain a large proportion of proteins but, except for the soybean, they do not contain all the essential amino acids. Vegetable proteins cannot replace the proteins of animal origin. However, vegetables (and fruits) are the main source, and in many cases the only source, of necessary vitamins and minerals. In addition, the fibers of vegetables (and fruits) promote intestinal motility and aid in the absorption and utilization of the nutrients. Regular consumption of vegetables is of foremost importance for maintaining good health, and nutritionists recommend that the daily diet should contain, besides starchy vegetables (e.g., potatoes, corn), leafy green and yellow vegetables. Since cooking destroys various nutrients (especially the water-soluble vitamins), or reduces their effectiveness, raw vegetables (e.g., salads) should be included in the diet. Organically grown vegetables are available in health food stores.

VEGETARIANISM

The theory and practice of living solely on foods of plant origin, that is, vegetables, fruits, grains (seeds), and nuts, and excluding from the diet all foodstuffs in any form that are of animal origin. There are the "lacto-ovo" (milk and eggs) vegetarians who exclude all flesh foods from the diet, but consume milk, eggs, butter, cheese, and other dairy products. Some vegetarians reject all flesh foods but will eat netted fish in addition to dairy products. There are also a comparatively few people, called the "fruitarians," who confine their diet to fruits only. It is known that the biologically most effective, or "complete" proteins are primarily in foods of animal origin. The intake of such proteins may, in addition, render inferior vegetable proteins more effective. Most nutritionists acknowledge that it is possible, though in some cases difficult, to obtain a balanced diet without flesh foods, but they maintain that complete abstinence from all foods of animal origin may cause nutritional deficiencies. It is pointed out that man is neither exclusively herbivorous nor carnivorous, but omnivorous. The practice of vegetarianism dates back many centuries and probably originated as a religious or humanitarian custom. There are several Hindu, Buddhist, and Christian sects, and followers of other teachings and beliefs who adhere to various forms of vegetarianism. As a movement concerned with nutrition rather than with religion and philosophy, vegetarianism became popular in the United States and in Europe around the middle of the last century. It is still practiced by many people, including well-known personalities in public life, the arts and professions.

VENISON (fr. OF *veneison* hunting, game, fr. L. *venari* to pursue, to hunt)

Originally the name applied to the edible parts of all game animals, such as deer, boar, pheasant, quail, but now restricted to the flesh of the animals belonging to the deer family (*Cervidae*), for example, the white-tailed, black-tailed, and mule deer, the reindeer, red deer, caribou, elk. In the Americas, Asia, and Europe, deer was hunted for its flesh which provided food, for its skin which was made into cloth, and for its antlers from which tools were carved. Venison is regarded by many people as a delicacy, particularly in Europe and Asia, and in certain parts of the world it is still a prime source of food. Venison tastes best when the animal is not too lean and over five years old. The distinctive taste and texture of the meat is greatly improved by "hanging" it for a few days in a cool and dry place. Hanging allows the formation of lactic acid which acts on the tissues, thereby increasing softness of the meat and enhancing its flavor. Venison is meat and as such contains all the nutrients indigenous to other types of meat. Since game animals inhabit areas which are remote from industries, where there are little or no agricultural activity, and feed on plants grown in soil usually free of chemical fertilizers and pesticides, advocates of natural foods consider venison (and other game meat) as a good source of clean, unadulterated meat.

VITAMINS (fr. L. *vita* life, and *amine* the name of a group of chemical compounds; originally it was believed that the vitamins belonged to these compounds; later this assumption was proven wrong, and the final e in the word *vitamine* was deleted)

General

The name of a group of unrelated organic substances that occur in small quantities in many foods, both of animal and plant origin, and are essential for the normal metabolic functioning of the body.

In 1897 a Dutch physician, Dr. Christian Eijkman, proved that the absence of a certain substance in the food can cause a severe disease, while the presence of that substance in the food can prevent and cure the same disease. This was confirmed in 1906 by an English biochemist, Sir Frederick G. Hopkins, who demonstrated that besides proteins, carbohydrates, and minerals, there are other substances necessary for health. They were called "accessory food factors." In 1912 a Polish (now American) biochemist, Dr. Casimir Funk, named these substances "vitamine" emphasizing that they are essential to life. He postulated the existence of other similar vital substances (vitamins B_1, B_2, C, and D). Since then many additional vitamins have been identified and synthetized.

Vitamins may be water-soluble or fat-soluble. Every vitamin has a very distinct function and cannot replace another, and all vitamins can be utilized effectively by the body only in the presence of minerals (e.g., calcium, phosphorus, iron, magnesium). Most vitamins are constantly being used as well as lost by excretion, and must be continuously replenished. Lack of the necessary amount of any vitamin in the daily diet may cause or prolong many disorders and diseases. If the diet does not provide the required vitamins in sufficient quantities, synthetized vitamins can be prescribed and taken orally or injected. There are also a great variety of vitamin preparations, extracted from natural sources, available as food supplements in health food stores.

For several vitamins a certain minimum daily requirement (MDR) has been set by the U.S. Government. There are a few vitamins for which the need in human nutrition has not been officially determined. Many scientists and nutritionists disagree with the Government's recommended minimum daily requirements and advocate higher amounts. They also claim that those vitamins for which the need has not been officially established are still essential to health. The vitamin content of the various foods and the daily requirements are measured and stated on the containers, for some vitamins in International Units (I.U.), and for some others in milligrams.

Vitamin A (carotene)

A fat-soluble vitamin which is stored in all fatty tissues. Vitamin A per se is not found in nature. It occurs as a "provitamin" only and its precursors are pigments (carotenoid substances, such as carotene) of plants. Vitamin A is formed from carotene in the liver of animals (including man). It is essential for maintaining good vision, and it is important for a healthy skin, the inner linings (mucous membranes) of the body, and for growth. Deficiency may cause growth retardation in children. Disturbed vision, especially night blindness and other eye diseases, roughness and dryness of the skin, toughening of the soft tissues, disturbances in digestion and reproductive functions are the results of vitamin A deficiency. Larger doses of vitamin A have been successfully used in the treatment of respiratory infections. However, prolonged intake of high doses of vitamin A can cause headache, nausea, and even enlargement of the liver and spleen, and fragility of the bones. The best sources of vitamin A are liver (e.g., fish, beef, chicken livers, cod or halibut liver oil), and other animal products (e.g., butter, cheese, milk), and yellow and leafy green vegetables (e.g., carrots, squash, sweet potatoes, kale, dandelion, corn). Vitamin A is easily destroyed in cooking, therefore, overcooking should be avoided. It is also susceptible to rapid deterioration if exposed to air. Freezing, however, does not significantly affect it. The recommended minimum daily allowance is 5,000 International Units for adults and teenagers, 6,000 to 8,000 for pregnant and nursing women. Many nutritionists suggest a daily intake of up to 20,000 International Units, not only because this amount is felt to be necessary for maintaining good health but also because it could increase longevity. (One cup of carrots contains about 15,000 I.U., three ounces of broccoli about 25,000 I.U., and four ounces of raw calf's liver about 25,000 I.U.)

Vitamin B complex

There are more than a dozen water-soluble substances identified in this group of vitamins. They cannot be stored in the body and must be replaced daily. Each member of the vitamin B complex has a distinct function, but all are interdependent. Most of these vitamins are found together in the same source but in different proportions. The effects of the B vitamins are very numerous. They are essential to the nervous and digestive systems, to the proper functioning of the heart and muscles, and they play a role in energy conversion and in the reduction of cholesterol accumulation.

Several substances, discovered in different countries at different times and identified as vitamins, were first designated as separate entities. Later research revealed that these substances actually belonged to the B group (e.g., vitamin G which is riboflavin or vitamin B_2). Some of the members of the B complex were then numbered, but some retained their chemical names. Not all of the B group have been found to play a role in human nutrition and they are therefore not usually included in the list of the B complex (e.g., B_3 which influences the growth of pigeon's feathers, B_4 which prevents a specific paralysis in rats and chicks).

Vitamin B_1 (thiamine hydrochloride)

The first vitamin to be discovered (in 1897) by a Dutch physician, Dr. Eijkman. He demonstrated that a widespread and often fatal disease (beriberi, fr. Singhalese "I am unable") affecting the people of the Far East and the East Indies, was due to the exclusive consumption of polished rice. The symptoms of the disease (e.g., extreme weakness, painful nerve inflammation, abnormal heart and digestive functions), disappeared when the diet contained unpolished (whole grain) rice. It was first believed that this was due to a single substance and was named later vitamin B, or antiberiberi factor. After many years of research, it was discovered that this vitamin can be divided into two different vitamins (B_1 and B_2, which made further divisions possible). Vitamin B_1 is vital to the normal activity of the nervous system and it is important in maintaining a balanced personality. It is required for orderly digestion, and it plays a role in the distribution of oxygen in the body. Deficiency in vitamin B_1 may lead to great weakness, various serious nervous disorders (e.g., neuralgia, insomnia), as well as to emotional instability. Best sources are whole grains and whole grain products, brewer's yeast, nuts, milk, lean pork, and liver. Vitamin B_1 is partially destroyed by cooking. The recommended daily allowance is approximately 1.2 to 1.5 milligrams. For people under stress or when very active, and also for the elderly, most nutritionists recommend higher doses and suggest a minimum daily intake of 10 milligrams. (Two tablespoons of brewer's yeast contain about 3 milligrams, one half of a cup of wheat germ about 1.5, and four ounces of calf's liver about 0.25.)

Vitamin B_2 (riboflavin)

It is important in the sugar and starch metabolism, and is needed for the oxygen exchange in the soft tissues. In combination with vitamin A, it promotes good vision, and protects the skin. Vitamin B_2 deficiency causes burning of the eyes. They become bloodshot and water readily, causing impaired vision. Lack of vitamin B_2 may lead to the development of cataracts. Sore lips and severe skin blemishes are the results of vitamin B_2 deficiency. The richest sources are organ meats (e.g., liver, heart, kidney), to a lesser degree lean meat and milk. Brewer's yeast and whole grains are good sources. Vitamin B_2 is less sensitive to heat than B_1, but it is quickly destroyed by sunlight. The recommended daily requirement is about 1.6 to 1.7 milligrams for men and 1.5 for women. This amount, however, is regarded by many nutritionists as far too low for optimum health, and they recommend a daily intake of at least 5 milligrams. (Four ounces of calf's liver contain about 4 milligrams, one cup of kidney stew about 2 milligrams, one half of a cup of wheat germ about 0.5 milligram.)

Vitamin B₆ (pyridoxine hydrochloride)

It occurs in the form of the phosphate in various animal and plant tissues and is important in the metabolism of proteins and in blood building. Vitamin B₆ enhances the utilization of fat and greatly influences the healthy functioning of the nerves and muscles. Deficiency may cause convulsion in infants. Skin disorders, sea-sickness, and dizziness may follow vitamin B₆ deficiency. In serious deficiency cases the body's ability to manufacture the blood protein hemoglobin is considerably impaired, thereby causing anemia. Vitamin B₆ is used in the treatment of various disorders of the nerves and muscles (e.g., cerebral palsy, epilepsy). Best sources are brewer's yeast, whole grains and whole grain products, organ meats (e.g., liver, kidney, brain), milk, egg yolk, cabbage, beets. Vitamin B₆ is not readily destroyed by heat, but meat products will lose up to 50 percent of their vitamin B₆ content if roasted or stewed. The required minimum daily amount has not been officially established; the National Academy of Science suggests between 0.53 to 1.21 milligrams. Some nutritionists, however, recommend a minimum daily intake of 2 to 5 milligrams.

Vitamin B_{12} (cyanocobalmin)

It has the most complex structure of all the known vitamins. Vitamin B_{12} is the only vitamin that contains a mineral (cobalt) and was originally called the "animal protein factor" because it was believed that it was obtainable from animal sources only. Vitamin B_{12} however is produced by various yeasts, especially as a by-product in streptomycin manufacture, and is now available in synthesized form. It protects the nerves against degeneration which usually occurs in severe anemias. It is one of the absolutely necessary substances for the proper production of blood. An infinitesimal amount is highly beneficial in combating pernicious anemia and in arresting deterioration of the cells of the central nervous system, as well as in reversing growth retardation in children. Vitamin B_{12} deficiency causes extreme weakness, pain, numbness of the arms and legs, enlargement of the liver, and may ultimately lead to death. Since it occurs in the liver and the muscles, the best sources are consequently the liver, lean meat, milk and milk products, and brewer's yeast. The minimum daily requirement has not been officially established, but an extremely small amount (i.e., 5 micrograms) is sufficient and effective.

Niacin (nicotinic acid)

There are actually two substances, niacin and niacinamide (nicotinamide) which, however, are usually listed together as niacin. They are also known as the P.P. vitamin (pellagra-preventing factor). Niacin dilates the blood vessels and increases the circulation, therefore, most vitamin supplements contain niacinamide which does not have these effects. Niacin was the first vitamin to be synthesized (in 1867), without it being recognized as a vitamin. It is needed for the nervous system, proper brain functioning, and healthy skin. Niacin is frequently called the "courage vitamin" because deficiency causes personality disturbances which manifest themselves in undue fear, suspicion, and depression. These are also the early symptoms of pellagra, a skin disease, caused by the lack of niacin in the diet. Severe deficiency may cause cessation of normal digestion, diarrhea, complete debilitation, and insanity. The best sources are liver, beefsteak, whole grains (rice, wheat), peanut, and brewer's yeast. Niacin is not destroyed by heat but it is lost into the cooking water. The recommended minimum daily requirement is 6 milligrams per 1,000 calories, or approximately 20 milligrams for an average daily intake of about 2,500 to 3,000 calories. Most nutritionists claim that an adult needs a daily intake of 30 to 100 milligrams. (Four ounces of beefsteak contain about 8.5 milligrams, two tablespoons of brewer's yeast about 10 milligrams, two ounces of raw beef liver about 15 milligrams.)

Pantothenic Acid

It occurs in all animal and plant tissues and is found in the cells of many microorganisms. It apparently influences the activity of the adrenal glands and affects the functioning of the entire alimentary canal. It was claimed that pantothenic acid plays a role in the prevention of early graying of hair and in the protection of the skin; these claims have not been substantiated by scientific evidence. It is used in the treatment of digestive disorders, and in conditions where there is a depressed function of the adrenal glands. The exact role of pantothenic acid in human nutrition, however, has not been firmly determined. Higher amounts of pantothenic acid in the daily diet proved to be beneficial in cases of stress and in increasing resistance to infections. The best sources are organ meats (e.g., liver, kidney), whole grains (e.g., rice, wheat), egg yolk, cabbage, broccoli. The daily requirement is unknown. Some nutritionists suggest a daily intake of up to 20 milligrams, especially in cases of serious injuries and burns.

Folic Acid

Together with vitamin B_{12} and vitamin C, it is essential for normal blood production. It influences the size and amount of the red blood cells. Folic acid deficiency causes anemia and contributes to liver dysfunction and digestive disturbances. It is used in the treatment of pernicious anemia, and in the correction of impaired fat metabolism. Folic acid is abundant in green leafy vegetables, in organ meats (e.g., liver, kidney), fresh mushrooms, brewer's yeast, whole grains and whole grain products. The required daily amount is unknown but most nutritionists agree that the average daily intake should be as high as 5 milligrams.

Para-amino-benzoic Acid

It influences the functioning of the endocrine glands and with other vitamins of the B complex (choline and pantothenic acid); it is used in restoring the original color of prematurely gray hair. It helps to restrain the overactivity of the thyroid glands and to normalize the function of the pituitary gland, thereby exerting a beneficial effect in rheumatoid arthritis. The need for para-amino-benzoic acid in human nutrition per se has not been established. It is actually part of the molecular structure of folic acid. It is found in all foods rich in the other vitamins of the B complex (e.g., organ meats, whole grains, brewer's yeast).

Choline

It is important in fat metabolism and in the proper functioning of the nervous system. Choline deficiency may cause accumulation of cholesterol, fatty degeneration of the liver, and impaired kidney function. Together with other vitamins of the B complex, it is used in the treatment of various liver disorders, glaucoma, and muscular dystrophy. The need for choline in human nutrition is recognized but the minimum daily requirement for it has not been established. The richest food sources for choline are liver, kidney, egg yolk, whole grains, and brewer's yeast.

Biotin

A very potent and widely distributed vitamin in animal and plant tissues. It is generally regarded as being vitally necessary for growth and good health. It functions in the metabolism of proteins, carbohydrates, and fats. Deficiency in biotin may lead to anemia, skin disorders, and sometimes to mental distress. However, only an extremely small amount is required and that is supplied in foods which contain the other members of the B complex. Therefore, a naturally occurring deficiency in biotin is very unlikely. It is found in organ meats (liver, kidney), in vegetables and nuts, brewer's yeast, and whole grains. The minimum daily requirement has not been established.

Inositol

The need for inositol in human nutrition has not been established but it is known that this vitamin (together with choline) plays a role in fat metabolism, especially in dissolving cholesterol. It occurs in the liver, brain, kidneys, and muscles, and it has been used in the treatment of certain mental disorders and in diseases affecting the functions of the nerves and muscles (e.g., muscular dystrophy, cerebral palsy), as well as in correcting hardening of the arteries. Inositol is present in most foods containing the other vitamins of the B complex (e.g., organ meats, whole grains), and in grapefruit, oranges, cantaloupe, and peas.

Several vitamins of the B complex (i.e., vitamin B_2, B_6, niacin, folic acid, and biotin) are also manufactured by various microorganisms (bacteria) which thrive in the intestines.

Vitamin C (ascorbic acid)

One of the most important vitamins since it aids the formation of collagen (an intercellular glue-like substance) that holds all cells of the body together. It is equally important in the development of healthy bones and teeth, and in keeping the connective tissues of the muscles firm. Without adequate supply of vitamin C, the bone-building minerals cannot perform properly. It also plays a role in the formation and maturation of red blood cells. It is known to increase resistance to shock and infections, although its precise role in such cases is not clearly understood. It is essential to the adrenal glands for producing cortisone (a hormone which has life-maintaining properties and important metabolic effects). Extreme vitamin C deficiency causes scurvy, a disease which results in bleeding of the gums and the small blood vessels into the tissues, anemia, general debility, and ultimately death. Scurvy was probably the first disease to be recognized as the consequence of nutritional deficiency. Since vitamin C is now the easiest to obtain of all vitamins, scurvy has become a rare disease. However, a milder form, due to vitamin C deficiency, causing small red spots on the skin formed by the bleeding of the small vessels, still affects many people. Vitamin C deficiency may result in loosening of the teeth, soreness of the joints, easy bleeding and bruising, slow healing of wounds, weak muscle functions, susceptibility to infections (especially to colds), loss of appetite and weight, general weakness, and irritability. Vitamin C in high doses is used as an adjuvant in the treatment of various disorders and diseases (e.g., febrile infections, poisoning), not necessarily directly connected to a deficiency.

Vitamin C is not stored in the body, and daily replacement is essential. Smoking tobacco and drinking alcoholic beverages increase the need for vitamin C considerably since tobacco and alcohol neutralize and destroy a large amount of it in the body. All fresh fruits and vegetables contain vitamin C in various amounts; it is also present in the liver, brain, and raw clams and oysters. It is very sensitive to heat, therefore uncooked (raw) fruits and vegetables (e.g., green peppers, tomatoes, cabbage, carrots) should be part of the daily diet. Since vitamin C dissolves in water, cooked vegetables should be served with the water. The recommended daily allowance is 60 milligrams for men and 55 milligrams for women. Pregnant and nursing women require higher amounts. Most nutritionists agree that these doses are far too low, especially during illness. They recommend a minimum daily intake of 200 to 300 milligrams. (One medium size orange contains about 50 milligrams, a green pepper about 100 milligrams, one half of a cup of rose hip, depending on the strength of the concentration, about 1,000 to 5,000 milligrams.)

The Bioflavonoids (formerly called Vitamin P)
A combination of several substances occurring in various fruits and plants (e.g., citrus fruits, Hungarian red pepper, red and black currants, rose hip). The bioflavonoids are important for reducing the fragility of the capillaries (small blood vessels), for increasing their strength and thereby protecting against viral invasion of the body. The use of bioflavonoids proved to be successful in the treatment of various types of bleedings, high blood pressure, and in the prevention of violent allergic reactions. They provide protection against a great number of ailments, such as stroke, rheumatoid arthritis, diabetes, cirrhosis of the liver, and are useful in averting respiratory infections, especially colds. The bioflavonoids play an important role in aiding the effectiveness of vitamin C and in protecting it from oxidation in the body. There is a definite interaction and interrelation between vitamin C and the bioflavonoids. The bioflavonoids are

not stored in the body and must be replaced daily. During illness and stress the need for them increases. Although the need for the bioflavonoids in human nutrition has not been officially established, most nutritionists agree that they are vital and must be supplied in the daily diet, and they suggest at least 200 to 300 units per day. The best sources are red and black currants, citrus fruits, green peppers, spinach, rose hip, asparagus, apricots, and lettuce. The bioflavonoids are destroyed when boiled or exposed to air. Sufficient consumption of raw fruits and vegetables is the best way to obtain the necessary supply. (One glass of orange juice contains about 500 international units, a half cup of spinach about 100 units, 100 grams of rose hip concentrate approximately 25,000 units.)

Vitamin D

There are actually two substances listed under vitamin D: one is calciferol (or D_2), the other is dehydrocholesterol (or D_3). Vitamin D is the only vitamin which is not found in foods of plant origin (except in a very minute quantity in mushrooms). It is essential in the assimilation of calcium and phosphorus in the body by activating the phosphatase (an enzyme) which aids the combination of phosphorus with calcium and their deposit in the bones and teeth. Vitamin D is important in helping to burn sugar efficiently, thereby releasing energy and preventing fatigue. It prevents rickets, a disease which results in deformed bone growth in children (e.g., bowlegs, knock knees, buck teeth), and in the weakening and softening of the bones of adults. Vitamin D in high doses is used in the treatment of arthritis. However, large amounts of this vitamin may sometimes have toxic effects (e.g., nausea, insoluble calcium deposits in the tissues, kidney damage). Deficiency may also cause flabby and weak muscle structure. Vitamin D is fat-soluble and it can be stored in the body but it is used up easily. Vitamin D_2 (calciferol) occurs in nature as ergosterol (a fatlike substance) in animal and plant tissues (e.g., in the oils of the human skin, in certain vegetable oils) and after exposure to sunshine (or when irradiated by ultraviolet rays, the artificial sunshine), it changes into the vitamin which can be utilized by the body. Vitamin D_3 (dehydrocholesterol) occurs in livers, especially in fish livers and fish liver oils, and to a lesser degree in other animal products. Actually, no foods per se can offer an adequate supply of vitamin D, therefore, regular exposure to sunshine whenever feasible is recommended. The best sources are fish liver oils and fortified milk, beef and chicken liver, egg yolk and butter. The recommended minimum daily requirement is 400 international units for infants and adults. Because of the possible toxic effects, larger doses should not be taken, especially by infants, without consulting a physician.

Vitamin E (tocopherol)

A group of related, fat-soluble substances consisting of at least six members of which the actions and effects of the alpha, beta, and gamma-tocopherols are the best known. The alpha form is the most effective. Vitamin E occurs naturally as a light yellow viscous oil. The exact role of vitamin E in human nutrition is not clear but it is generally agreed that man requires this vitamin. It is stored mainly in the pituitary, adrenal, and sex glands. It is essential for normal reproduction in some animals, and is believed to have the same function in humans. Miscarriages have been traced to vitamin E deficiency, and it has been used for the prevention of spontaneous abortion and in the correction of impaired fertility. Vitamin E has been successfully employed in the treatment of cardio-vascular diseases, multiple sclerosis and other neuromuscular conditions, arthritis, and mental disorders. Since it is fat-soluble, disturbances in fat metabolism may obstruct the utilization of vitamin E in the body. Vitamin E aids in supplying oxygen to the cells, and it enhances the detoxification process in the liver. Rancid fats as well as food refining processes destroy it but cooking does not. The best sources are wheat germ, vegetable oils, beef liver, cod liver oil, eggs, soybean, kale, and turnip. The National Research Council suggested that the vitamin E requirement may be between 25 to 30 milligrams depending on the fat consumed. It is known that the requirement for vitamin E increases if the total fat intake consists of more than 20 percent of polyunsaturated fats. Most nutritionists recommend a daily minimum intake of 50 to 100 milligrams. (One ounce of wheat germ contains about 110 milligrams, three ounces of beef liver about 1.4 milligrams, one half of a cup of raw wheat germ about 30 milligrams.)

Vitamin K

Two related substances that are essential for the formation of prothrombin, a blood-clotting enzyme which prevents abnormal bleeding. K_1, an oily substance, is obtained from plant sources, and K_2, a crystalline substance, is produced by microorganisms. K_2 is also synthetized by intestinal bacteria. Both forms of the vitamin K are now derived from mendione (a simple organic matter) which has a more effective blood-clotting potency than the natural vitamin. Vitamin K (natural or synthetized) is, however, ineffective in hemophilia (a hereditary disease affecting almost exclusively the male and causing uncontrollable bleeding). Vitamin K, like the other fat-soluble vitamins (A, D, and E), requires fat intake and bile salts in order to be absorbed and utilized by the body. A deficiency considerably prolongs the time needed for normal blood-clotting, thereby causing abnormal bleeding. It is used as a preventative in various operations, in labor, and wherever strong bleeding is anticipated. Vitamin K is usually not sufficiently active in the blood of new born infants and therefore in such cases vitamin K injections are administered. The need for vitamin K in human nutrition and the minimum daily requirement have not been determined. Deficiency in this vitamin is very rarely of dietary origin. Many leafy green vegetables (e.g., cabbage, spinach), liver, and egg yolk contain sufficient amounts of vitamin K. It is not readily destroyed by heat.

Synthetic Vitamins (fr. Gk. *syn* together and *tithenial* to put)

Vitamins artificially produced by chemical synthesis, that is, not extracted from natural sources (plants, animals). Synthetic vitamins are identical with, and have the same effects as those occurring in nature. There are, however, many yet unknown and/or unsynthetized substances present in natural sources that are essential as complementary factors for the proper utilization of other nutrients. Therefore, in certain cases, synthetic vitamins would not suffice (e.g., a synthetic vitamin C tablet usually does not contain the bioflavonoids which protect it from oxidation in the body).

WATER

Regular

A tasteless, odorless, transparent liquid, which, colorless in smaller amounts, has a bluish, greenish tint in large quantities. Chemically, it is a compound of hydrogen and oxygen. When water is cooled to its freezing temperature (32° F or 0° C), it becomes solid (ice) and, unlike other liquids, it expands; when exposed to ordinary temperature it eventually evaporates, and when heated to its boiling point (212° F or 100° C), it vaporizes to steam. About 70 percent of the earth's surface is covered by water (the oceans, lakes, streams, and glaciers). Life on earth originated in water, and without water there would be no life. Of all inorganic compounds present in the protoplasm (the fundamental substance of which all living matter is composed), water is the most important and most abundant. The human body consists primarily of water (about 65 percent). Water is one of the best solvents; it dissolves and mixes more substances than any other liquid, thus it keeps suspended, carries, and disperses all organic and inorganic matters which are essential to maintaining and sustaining life of animals and plants.

The average fluid intake of a moderately active healthy person is about 5.5 pints of which approximately 3 pints are water and beverages, and 2.5 pints are obtained from solid foods (e.g., fruits, vegetables, lean meat), and from liquid foods (e.g., milk, soups). These 5.5 pints of the normal daily water intake are eliminated mostly as urine (about 60 percent), sometimes as undetectable perspiration (about 25 percent), as vapor in the air exhaled from the lungs (about 12 percent), and in the feces (about 3 percent). The body requires more fluid intake if there is a greater loss of water through excessive perspiration due to hot weather or overactivity. Such losses should be replaced and, because sweat contains salt, physicians also recommend replacing the salt. Contrary to certain beliefs, water is not harmful to health, except when it is impure or contaminated. It is generally contraindicated in some diseases (e.g., various heart conditions, kidney inflammation) where reduction of the water intake is advised; in certain other illnesses (e.g., kidney stones, gout) the intake of excess water is sometimes part of the treatment. However, claims that it is necessary to drink large amounts of water and other fluids to remain healthy, to wash out poisonous wastes, or to cleanse the intestines have no scientific validity. In various infectious and febrile diseases (e.g., common cold), an increase in the fluid intake is usually recommended. Under normal conditions excessive thirst or increased elimination of water may be signs of serious disorders.

Many health food advocates recommend drinking and using for cooking bottled (spring) waters instead of ordinary tap water.

Mineral Waters

Spring waters containing various mineral salts (e.g., carbonates, chlorides, silicates), and metallic sulfates (e.g., calcium, iron, magnesium) in sufficient quantities to give the waters special properties and taste, and to render them useful as adjuvants in the treatment of various diseases. Several of the mineral waters contain naturally occurring gases (e.g., the effervescent spring water in Niederselters, Germany; hence the name "seltzer water"), or are charged with carbon dioxide (e.g., the common soda water and the sparkling drinks). Spring waters containing iron salts and carbon dioxide are known as chalybeate waters (fr. L. *chalybs* steel).

Mineral waters are considered to be of value either in the direct treatment or in the prevention of a great variety of diseases and disorders, such as kidney and liver ailments, conditions of the digestive system, rheumatism, gout, diabetes and so forth. Drinking of mineral waters and bathing in the hot (thermal) springs for therapeutic purposes have been popular since ancient times in many parts of the world, especially in Europe. Today, the best known mineral waters are produced in France, Germany, Czechoslovakia, Hungary, and Poland where the bottling and marketing of these mineral waters is an important industry. The famous European spas, such as Aix-les-Bains (France), Baden-Baden (Germany), Carlsbad (Czechoslovakia), and Budapest (Hungary), attract many visitors every year. There are also several well-known mineral springs in the United States, such as Saratoga Springs, New York, White Sulphur Springs, West Virginia, Las Vegas Hot Springs, New Mexico, and Hot Springs, Arkansas. Springs producing mineral waters are mostly artesian wells (fr. *Artesium,* the Latin name of an ancient region in Northern France). In such wells the water is pushed upward through fissures by deep underground pressure and arrives at the surface through natural openings such as a fountain. Where the geological formation prevents the upward flowing of the water, artesian wells are created by drillings. Waters coming from very deep layers are usually warm or hot. Some mineral waters are manufactured synthetically by adding mineral to ordinary water in the same proportion as they occur in the natural spring waters. In many countries plain or effervescent spring waters with slight mineral content are used regularly as table water. Domestic and imported mineral waters are available in better groceries and in most health food stores.

Spring Waters

Waters which have accumulated in underground rocks and flow to the surface. In a stricter sense, such waters are not considered to be mineral waters though they do contain small amounts of various minerals. Most spring waters are slightly alkaline. They are free from organic impurities and taste better than ordinary drinking water but do not have direct therapeutic effects as some of the mineral waters have. The drinking of spring waters instead of ordinary water has always been common in many countries, particularly in Europe. The continuous treatment of ordinary water with chemicals in order to render it safe for human consumption usually results in an unsavory taste, but many people regard the use of chemicals in water as detrimental to health in other ways. In addition, the spreading awareness of the industrial pollution of soil and water resources has recently made the use of spring waters for drinking and cooking more popular in the United States. A great variety of spring waters, in glass bottles or plastic containers, are available in health food stores and practically in every grocery shop.

WHEAT

An annual cereal (grain) plant of the Grass family. It was probably the first domesticated and cultivated food plant of man. Grown in Egypt before 5000 B.C., it was introduced to Mesopotamia and India around 4000 B.C., and to China around 2500 B.C. From the Mediterranean regions, wheat spread to Western and Northern Europe where it was cultivated as far back as 2000 B.C. The civilizations of Europe and West Asia were based largely on wheat. Bread as a symbol of the divine Providence, as the representative of all foods and many times of life itself was incorporated into many beliefs and religious rites. Wheat became one of the most important food resources of the Western world. Today, the major wheat producing countries of the world are the United States, the USSR, China, Canada, India, Argentina, and Europe and Australia.

The ancestors of wheat are not precisely known. Modern wheat (*Triticum aestivum*) is classified according to planting seasons as winter (hard) and spring wheats. (The winter variety contains a high percentage of gluten, a proteinlike substance which makes the bread dough cohesive, and in extracted form gluten is used in bakery products for diabetics). Another wheat variety is durum (*Triticum durum*), which has the hardest kernels and is very rich in gluten. Its flour is used mainly in the production of spaghetti, macaroni, and other similar products. As bread flour, it is used mainly in India and China. The vegetative parts of wheat, and the by-products of milling, are used as livestock feed. Wheat is also used in the manufacture of alcoholic beverages, such as whisky, beer, and vodka. Practically every wheat-growing country carries out extensive research toward creating new varieties or improving existing ones in order to obtain greater yield, toward increasing the nutritional values, intensifying disease resistance properties, and to enhancing acclimatization to different environments. New and better varieties have already been produced successfully. Wheat flour is a highly nutritious product. If, however, in the milling and refining process the bran and the germ of the whole grain (which contains the valuable nutrients) are discarded, the flour is almost pure starch and is devoid of significant nutritional value. See: **Bran, Grain, Wheat Germ,** the subentry on Wheat Germ Oil under **Fats and Oils.**

WHEAT GERM

The wheat germ (embryo) constitutes only about 2 percent of the grain but nutritionally it is the most important part of it. The germ oil, the richest known source of the reproductive and growth factor, the vitamin E complex, also contains several vitamins of the B complex, vitamin A, and fatty acids. When the germ is ground into flour, the oils containing vitamin E combine with oxygen and may quickly become rancid, thereby destroying much of the vitamin E. Health food stores carry freshly milled, highly nutritious wheat germs as a food supplement, mostly in vacuum-packed containers which should be kept tightly covered and refrigerated. See: Subentries on Wheat Germ Oil, Vegetable Oils under **Fats and Oils.**

WHEY

The watery part of the milk (milk serum) left after the coagulable part, the protein-rich (casein) curd, is separated in the process of making cheese. It consists of water, soluble minerals, some fats, and it is rich in lactose and lactalbumin (another milk protein). Formerly, whey was wasted or else mixed into livestock feed, but now it is condensed and added to processed cheeses in order to augment their nutritional qualities. (In Scandinavia, whey is made into a special cheese.) Whey, in dried and pulverized form, is also used in various products providing nutritional food supplements, such as wafers and cookies, mostly mixed with other substances (e.g., bone meal, carob powder), or in paramedical preparations for digestion regulation, alone or mixed with thickening substances, such as pectin, guar gum. Several whey preparations, in powder and tablet forms, are available in health food stores. See: **Cheese.**

WHOLE FOODS

A name, generally applied by health food advocates to all unadulterated foodstuffs which have their natural nutritive values and are free of artificial (chemical) additives. For example, certified raw milk is considered as "whole food" as opposed to commercially processed milk, which is free of chemical additives, but in which the nutrients have been changed or decreased through pasteurization and homogenization; or, while the enriched whole grain bread does contain sufficient nutrients, it is not considered as "whole food" because it usually has added chemical preservatives to retard spoilage. See: **Health Foods, Natural Foods, Organic Foods.**

WILD RICE (also called water oats, Indian rice, Canada rice)

A tall, annual aquatic North American plant (*Zizania aquatica*) of the Grass family, yielding very nutritious edible seeds that somewhat resemble rice. Wild rice, however, does not belong to the same genus as the common (Asiatic) rice. The seeds once served as the main food for several Indian tribes. It grows in shallow waters and is an important source of food and shelter for fish and water fowl. It has never been cultivated with success, and the seeds for human consumption are still gathered by primitive methods. Wild rice contains more proteins and is richer in several vitamins of the B complex than the unpolished (brown) rice.

The marketed seeds are unprocessed and unpolished. Wild rice is available in health food stores and in better groceries.

YEAST

The common name of a great variety of microscopic fungi of the genus *Saccharomyces*. Yeasts are oval or round unicellular organisms that reproduce by detachment from each other (gemmation). The capability of yeast to bring about chemical changes (fermentation, leavening) in certain foods and drinks, has been utilized for centuries, especially in making alcoholic beverages and bread. In breadmaking, the yeast affects the carbohydrate sugar content of the dough by changing it into carbon dioxide, the gas which causes the dough to rise, and ethyl alcohol, which evaporates during baking and creates the pleasant odor characteristic of bakeries and freshly baked products. It was believed for a long time that yeasts possessed therapeutic properties and they were used in the treatment of various ailments. Later it was found that many yeasts are actually pathogenic for men and animals. However, there is a yeast obtained as a by-product of the beer-brewing process that, because of its high nutrient content, is considered as a useful food supplement, especially in cases of vitamin B deficiency. Nutrients in the fresh yeast used for leavening bread dough and other flour products cannot be utilized by the human body and, contrary to some popular beliefs, its consumption will not correct nutritional deficiencies or cure disease. In certain cases, eating baker's yeast may cause adverse reactions. See: **Additives, Leavening Agents, Brewer's Yeast.**

YOGURT (yoghurt, fr. Tk. *yoğurt*)

A semisolid food made of the cow's or goat's whole or skimmed milk by fermentation with lactic acid producing microorganisms, especially *Lactobacillus bulgaricus.* Yogurt has always been part of the regular daily diet of the peoples of the Balkan States. The Russian zoologist, Elie Metchnikoff (1845–1916), after studying the longevity and remarkable good health of many Bulgarian farmers and herdsmen, attributed these phenomena to the regular consumption of large quantities of yogurt. His findings, published at the end of the last century (and later corroborated to a certain degree by other investigators) made yogurt a popular food supplement in Europe. Yogurt is rich in predigested proteins, in vitamins B_1 and B_2 (it also "creates" them for future use), and establishes an acid medium in the intestinal tract in which minerals are easily absorbed but which inhibits the growth of harmful and putrefaction causing bacteria. In this respect, it is superior to sour milk, and is digested faster and better than ordinary milk. Yogurt is available plain or mixed with fruits. Health food stores carry plain yogurt, or mixed with natural vanilla, made from certified raw milk. Cultures for making yogurt at home are also available. See: Subentries on Fermented Milk, Certified Raw Milk under Milk.